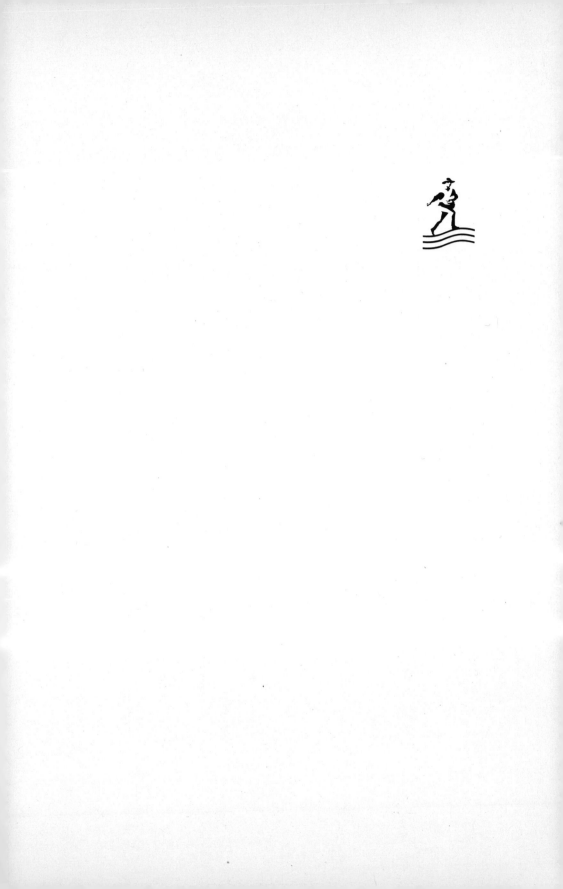

Last
Acts

Discovering Possibility and
Opportunity at the End of Life

DAVID J. CASARETT, M.D.

SIMON & SCHUSTER
New York   London   Toronto   Sydney

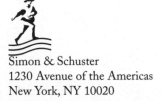

Simon & Schuster
1230 Avenue of the Americas
New York, NY 10020

First Simon & Schuster hardcover edition January 2010

SIMON & SCHUSTER and colophon are registered trademarks of Simon & Schuster, Inc.

For information about special discounts for bulk purchases, please contact Simon & Schuster Special Sales at 1-866-506-1949 or business@simonandschuster.com

The Simon & Schuster Speakers Bureau can bring authors to your live event. For more information or to book an event contact the Simon & Schuster Speakers Bureau at 1-866-248-3049 or visit our website at www.simonspeakers.com.

Designed by Jaime Putorti

Manufactured in the United States of America

10 9 8 7 6 5 4 3 2 1

Library of Congress Cataloging-in-Publication Data
Casarett, David J.
    Last acts : discovering possibility and opportunity at the end of life / David J. Casarett.
        p. cm.
    Includes bibliographical references and index.
    1. Terminal care—Case studies. 2. Terminally ill—Psychology
3. Death. 4. Quality of life. I. Title.
    R726.8.C397 2010
    616'.029—dc22   2009016590
ISBN: 978-1-4165-8037-9

CONTENTS

CONTENTS

For my father, Louis J. Casarett (1927–1972)

Last
Acts

For the most part, this book is comprised of stories that tend to speak for themselves. They don't need much preparation or explanation, and in fact I've chosen them precisely because they stand on their own so well. That is, they demand little of me, and that is a quality that struck me—a first-time author—as being invaluable. There are, however, two things I should say about these stories that will provide a useful context.

The first is an explanation—a map, really—of the origins of these stories. Physicians have won a generally well-deserved reputa tion as a conservative lot, averse to novelty and change and ponderously adherent to tradition. But in one respect at least, geographically, we're actually quite liberated, even nomadic. Medical education usually comprises college in one city, followed by medical school in another, and so on through an endless series of cheap apartments—which we never see—as we make our sleep-deprived way through internship, residency, and fellowships.

My own career has been no exception, and these stories come from several stops along that journey. A handful, for instance, are taken from my days as a medical student at Case Western Reserve University in Cleveland. For four years I bounced back and forth across Euclid Avenue from the hospitals on one side of the street, where my clinical responsibilities lay, to graduate school in medical anthropology, where I found a strange sort of intellectual respite from the routine and rote memorization of medical school. From Cleveland, I went on to do a residency in internal medicine at the University of Iowa, and it was during my training there, and a subsequent chief residency, that I met the patients in the first three chapters—Jacob, Danny, and Alberto.

I spent a wonderful year, next, at the University of Chicago doing a fellowship in medical ethics, where I met Marie, in chapter 5. From there I came to the University of Pennsylvania to do a fellowship with my mentor, Dr. Janet Abrahm, and it was during that fellowship that I met Tom (chapter 6) and Lacy (chapter 7). After my fellowship, I stayed at the University of Pennsylvania and at the Philadelphia VA Medical Center, where my clinical work is based. And it was through my work there that I met Ladislaw (chapter 8) and Jose (chapter 9). Finally, my work as a researcher has given me a chance to meet people all over the country and indeed around the world, and I met Christine, the subject of chapter 10, during one such trip.

Each of these stories is based on my recollections of patients I've taken care of. That is, the main themes of each are true, at least as true as memory permits. But these stories are faithful only within the bounds of the infidelities of memory. Some characters are composites, and dialogue is necessarily recreated. The stories are, I suppose, less reconstructions than they are re-creations.

Although I had anticipated and accepted this necessity when I began to write, there was another difficulty that I hadn't fully appreciated. In sketching the outlines of these stories I found myself worrying about what families might think if they were to read them. (My belief that this book would be read widely enough to create such a risk was surely a delusion, but such delusions are, of course, an author's prerogative).

I worried, for instance, that many of these stories would divulge details about a patient that families might not have known. And that they might include details that the patient would not have wanted their families to learn. I worried, too, about those stories in this collection—many of them—that offer my own interpretation of a patient's motivations and goals. It might be inappropriate, I thought, to reinterpret events years after my patient died and families had made their peace.

So in re-creating these stories I've adhered to the conventions of medical case reports in the scientific literature that require details about the patients to be omitted, obscured, or altered. I've changed all of their names, for instance, and many of their details. And I've either omitted or changed the names of some locations that would offer clues to the patient's identity. Finally, I've omitted or altered the names of physicians, nurses, and others for whom these patients would be easily recognizable. For patients, I've used only a first name, which is a pseudonym. In some cases I've used actual names because these people deserve credit for their roles as colleagues, mentors, or friends.

So these stories are not factually accurate. Unless, of course, the tricks of memory have somehow conspired with the process of concealment to bring these accounts full circle, making them more true than I intended. Nevertheless, I'm confident that they capture the essence of the people they describe and, even more important, their motivations.

Sylvester

Sylvester

It was when I was finishing rounds in my hospital late one evening that I first began to think about how my patients should spend their time when that time was cruelly limited. I'd just spent what felt like hours trying unsuccessfully to wrap up a difficult conversation with Sylvester, an older man who had a particularly vicious form of renal cancer. That his cancer was so extensive when it was discovered was due at least in part to a colleague's talent for inventing benign explanations for the increasingly numerous symptoms that Sylvester brought to clinic every month. My colleague dismissed Sylvester's symptoms first as "nerves" and later as "old age" until they were explained, finally, by the cancer that would kill him.

This was the second time that Sylvester and I had met, and again our conversation quickly descended into a protracted and dispiriting review of Sylvester's treatment options, which were limited, and the chance of success with each, which was essentially zero. We had been talking for well over an hour about his cancer, possible treatments, and even experimental protocols for which he wouldn't have been eligible anyway. The conversation had become like a juggling act in which clubs were replaced by phrases—"quality of life," "comfort care," "aggressive treatment"—that he and I tossed back and forth until, for me at least, they had lost their meaning. In fact, I'm not sure these terms ever had much meaning for Sylvester. His mind was clearly elsewhere, and that night, just as he had during our first visit, he kept circling back to his missed diagnosis with a predictability that was becoming disheartening.

It had grown dark outside his hospital room, which was itself lit only by a pale, flickering fluorescent tube on the wall just above Sylvester's head. The hospital ward had grown quiet, and even the shouts and metallic hammering of the construction site across 38th Street had been replaced by an eerie silence. And any remaining hope I had for a resolution to our discussion disappeared as I realized that Sylvester, who was Italian, began to lose his already tenuous grasp on English grammar and pronunciation as he became more emotional. He was working himself into a fit over his mistreatment, and our discussion swirled around and around, propelled by language that bore a diminishing resemblance to English.

Finally, though, despite many misunderstandings, we seemed to be making progress across a river of circular arguments and recriminations. But just when I thought we had succeeded in hauling each other out of the other side, Sylvester stopped me with a question that sent us right back to where we started: "What I do now?"

I shrugged—what choice did I have?—and waded back into a discussion of treatment options. But he stopped me again, in English that was suddenly so clear it was hard to imagine our past hour of missed communication and said, "No. No, I mean, I have no time left. What I do?"

I wish I could say that this question—the most significant one he had asked me in our short but intense relationship—led to a meaningful discussion and let us connect as we hadn't before. But no, I dodged it. Just as most doctors would, I think.

How should Sylvester spend the rest of his life? What sort of a question is that for a physician? He should ask his wife, perhaps, or their children. Or his priest. Or maybe this question was something he just needed to work out for himself. But I was stunned that he would ask me.

I was also reluctant to answer because I was, suddenly, in new territory for which I didn't have a map. And that is anxiety-provoking for any physician, and particularly for one who was as young as I was then. I thought I would say the wrong thing, and that I might tell Sylvester what he didn't want to hear. Or worse, that I would give him advice—the wrong advice—that he would accept.

Mostly, though, I think I was reluctant to offer an answer because Sylvester's question was so intensely personal. An answer, if I'd been prepared to offer one, would have implied a rich appreciation of his life that I didn't have, and indeed would never have. And his question seemed to imply that he wanted to establish the relationship that my answer would require. It was almost as if he were saying, "OK, it's so easy for you to talk *to* me with rehearsed answers about treatment. Here's a question that will force you to talk *with* me." It created a forced, importuning intimacy that I wasn't comfortable accepting, and an intimacy for which I hadn't yet mastered the physician's dubious skill of avoiding gracefully.

I'm not sure what I told Sylvester that night: "Whatever you want," or maybe "Whatever you think is most important to you." I don't know what advice I offered, if I offered any at all, but it was probably as thin and weak as the hospital vending-machine coffee he used to complain about. I do know, though, that his question evaporated as I left the hospital and walked down an empty Market Street that night in time to catch the last train home.

Last Acts

But ideas—at least important ones—are persistent. They may disappear, leaving you alone for a while, but they eventually come back again, and again, until you pay attention to them. This is fortunate, because I suspect that most of us can't be trusted to recognize an important idea the first time it comes calling.

I wish I could point to an epiphany of my own that led me to return to Sylvester's question with the intensity that would make a book worthwhile. That would make for a convincing story, but unfortunately it's not true. The truth, as far as I can discern it, is that this book is the product of an endless series of nudges, increasing in frequency and intensity, which have propelled me from that evening visit to Sylvester's hospital room to this book.

That his question stayed with me is due largely to my patients. I'm a palliative-care physician, and so most of my patients are near the end of life. Many have several months to live but some, when I meet them, only have a few days or hours. And all of them, no matter how little time they have left, and no matter what their background, have answered Sylvester's question in their own ways. A few, as Sylvester did, have made the mistake of asking me for advice. But most, fortunately, seem to know better and turn elsewhere. Still, I heard Sylvester's question, or variants of it, often enough that I gradually began to pay attention.

And once I did, I began to see Sylvester's question everywhere. In the multiple tragedies of September 11, 2001, for instance. And the Sago mining disaster, and the sinking of the Russian submarine *Kursk*. All of these events and many more have forced a wide variety of people to recognize, often with tragic suddenness, that they have very little time left. Some—the fortunate ones, perhaps—have a chance to ask the same question that Sylvester asked me: "What should I do with the time I have left?" And a few—the very lucky few—have time to find an answer and to act.

The result, for these victims of tragedies and for my patients, is the last acts that fill whatever time they have. Some last acts are so small as to be barely noticeable, and vanish into the swirl of emotion and activity that surround a death. Notes to family members, for instance, or small changes to a will. Others are the product of grand efforts—novels, films, works of art—that leave a lasting mark. But I began to see that I could learn from all of them.

A Lady in Hyde Park

Visitors to my office are often impressed by the photographs that hang on the walls. It's a collection, mostly, of large framed color photographs that I've taken and sold over the years, to support my university's partnership with an AIDS hospice in Botswana. So visitors exclaim over my amateurish photographs of children and all manner of wildlife, and occasionally even purchase one, sending a few dollars to people in Africa whom they'll never meet.

But there is one photograph, hanging over my desk, which they seem to miss. Much smaller than its neighbors, it's in black and white. It seems to be hiding, unwilling to compete with its bright, oversized neighbors.

The photo frames an elderly woman in profile, resting on a park bench in London's Hyde Park. Both of her hands are tightening her collar against what I imagine to be a cold London spring day, giving her an attitude that, at first glance, looks like prayer. Her feet are extended delicately along the length of a cane that is propped on the edge of the bench in an artful arrangement that succeeds in seeming both clever and perfectly natural. The few visitors who do notice it mistakenly assume that it is my own work. No one yet has recognized it as one of the lesser-known photographs of the French photographer Henri Cartier-Bresson.

What impressed me about that photograph when I first saw it years ago, and what induced me to pay far too much for an original print in a gallery in Milan, was the graceful ease of the woman's position within the frame. She doesn't appear to be particularly fashionable, or elegantly dressed, and she is, after all, merely sitting on a park bench. Yet somehow out of that moment she has created a pose that succeeds in being both perfectly poised and—what is infinitely more difficult—perfectly natural.

Even more striking than her pose, though, is the mental attitude that brought her to that position at that moment. There is an attitude of what I read as comfortable resignation that seems to cradle and inspire her. Her image suggests to me an earlier hidden moment—a minute or an hour before Cartier-Bresson passed by—when circumstances led her to that bench. Perhaps her walk was to have taken her further into the park, to Speaker's Corner or around the Serpentine, and she became tired. Others no doubt paused at that bench that day, but they did so, I imagine, with a migratory tentativeness—touching down, gathering strength or breath—and moving on. But perhaps she paused for a moment, and the path leading onward disappeared. And it was then that she would have realized that this bench could be her stage, if she wanted it to be.

Although Cartier-Bresson is often credited with having an eye for the "decisive moment" when light and form come into perfect alignment, I'd prefer to give credit for this particular photograph to the unnamed woman herself. I'd like to believe that she recognized the challenge that her minor stage posed, and that she realized she could make something of this opportunity that would be uniquely hers, yet also graceful and natural enough to attract the lens of the passing photographer. And I'd like to think that she took stock of her limited props and decided that she could transform them into a pose that would be a work of art.

It doesn't matter to me that this story of mine is purely speculative. What is important to me, and why Cartier-Bresson's photograph hangs over my desk, is that the woman's attitude of creative pragmatism that I've conjured up is one that many of my patients need to adopt, whether they realize it or not. Like her, they've all come to a moment at which their lives are made of—and therefore must be made from—a much reduced set of props and materials. Instead of years ahead, filled with family, career, and friends, their future has been truncated by illness. And just as Cartier-Bresson's lady finds her life framed for a moment by that bench, my patients find their lives framed by whatever time—months or weeks or days—that they have left.

As Sylvester had, many of my patients try to fill that frame they're given with a picture that is uniquely their own. Sometimes their efforts produce a fine image—meticulously arranged and perfectly exposed—that will leave a lasting and treasured impression on all of us. But often the image that takes shape is one of fumbling trial and error, less like a fine silver gelatin print that belongs in a gallery and more like a snapshot captured at a family gathering.

Nevertheless, even when their compositions are slightly askew and out of focus, and even when they're populated with grinning awkwardness, these snapshots that describe my patients' last acts are still the genuine products of aspiration. All of them reveal a version of Sylvester's desire to fill a moment with the grace that Cartier-Bresson's lady achieved so effortlessly. So I don't find my patients' last acts any less compelling if they fall short of what they could have accomplished. In fact, I find that my attention is caught and held simply by the efforts of those, like Sylvester, who wanted to make something of the time that they have left.

A Taxonomy of Last Acts

This, then, was the frame in which Sylvester found himself an unwilling subject. But what were his options? What could he have done? As I left Sylvester's room that night and made my way home, I began to realize that I didn't have any idea.

What do we do when we know, or think, that we're going to die soon? Do we become more altruistic? Do we seek revenge? Do we seek pleasure, or forgiveness, or spiritual fulfillment?

I've seen these responses and many more in my own practice, and the possibilities seem endless. But I began to wonder whether maybe these possibilities are circumscribed by boundaries and categories. Maybe there is an overarching organizational structure—a taxonomy—of the last acts that people pursue near the end of life.

So that's partly what this book is about—a search for some set of organizing principles that lets us understand what we do when we're faced with death.

The stories that make up this book seem to have sorted themselves, through some organic process that I'm not sure I can explain, into one such taxonomy. It's certainly not the only one that can be imposed on a universe of stories and examples with such protean manifestations. But it is one taxonomy that has helped me to make sense of what we do and, more importantly, what we can do, when our time is limited.

The result is a collection of ten chapters and about fifty stories that I hope impose some sense and structure on the breadth of what's possible. These represent categories of last acts that Sylvester might have considered for himself. And, I suppose, they're the categories that I should have laid out for him that night.

For instance, I've begun by describing one patient in the first chapter who was less than a day away from death when I met him. Yet Jacob never seemed to consider the question that Sylvester had asked of me, nor did he do anything with the time he had left. At least he didn't do anything differently. His goal—his only goal, as near as I could tell—was to cling to life as long as possible. And although his striving won him a few more hours of life, he lost forever the chance to spend time with his family and to say goodbye to his fiancée. That chapter is my latest effort, one of many, to figure out why he was blind to the opportunities, which I saw so clearly, to make use of his time. And it is, too, a meditation on the line that separates people like Jacob who chase survival with a single-minded intensity from those, like Sylvester, who turn instead to consider how they can best use the time that they have left.

In a way, I suppose, the nine chapters that follow have a remedial tone. They're about people who did what Jacob wouldn't, or couldn't. They're stories of people who saw—more or less clearly—that their time was limited. And they all made a conscious effort to use that time for a purpose. That is, like Sylvester, they saw the opportunity that Jacob couldn't see. These are the stories and examples that I should have shared with Sylvester that night.

Sometimes these stories reflect purposes that were admirable, and which led to actions that most of us might do well to emulate. These patients of mine reconnected with friends and family, for instance (chapter 3), or made amends (chapter 4) or left a legacy (chapter 7), or helped others (chapter 8). Some examples are less grand but no less admirable (chapters 6 and 10). And at least one describes a course that I wouldn't recommend (chapter 9). Still others are more nuanced and defy snap judgments. Seeking pleasure, for instance (chapter 2) and seeking revenge (chapter 5) aren't wholly admirable, yet their imperfection makes them compelling.

But this book isn't only a balance sheet of good choices, because who of us, really, has made choices that would stand up to that sort of audit? It is, instead, an exploration of why people make the choices they do. It is, too, an exploration of the factors that make a particular choice right for one person and wrong for another.

Learning from Last Acts

As these stories assembled themselves into chapters, I realized that they offer more than a map of what's possible. Not only did these stories suggest options—options that I could have offered to Sylvester—they also raised questions. Questions I wanted to answer, and assumptions I wanted to test.

I wondered, for instance, how many people take the time to ask the question that Sylvester had asked of me. I wanted to believe that every one of us will devote as much attention as Sylvester did to making the most of whatever time we have left. But will we?

And I wondered, too, how many people ask Sylvester's question with the same intensity that he did. Sylvester had been a mason who had contributed to many of the homes in Philadelphia, and I could imagine him surveying the last weeks of his life that stretched out in front of him with the same critical attention that he would have devoted to a partially finished wall. I could imagine him squinting a bit, head cocked to one side, testing his trajectory against an invisible plan and rearranging his remaining days as he might have shifted stones into place, seeking the best fit and the truest line. But how many of us will take the measure of our remaining time with the same ponderous scrutiny?

And I was curious, too, about why we make the choices that we do. Why does one woman with cancer devote her final months to raising money for cancer research while another writes a brief autobiography to pass on to children and grandchildren? And why does one man in a hijacked plane join the struggle against the hijackers while the man next to him uses those last few minutes to send a message to his wife?

Finally, I wondered about the impact of these last acts on others. A skeptic might say that any such act is little more than a distraction. That is, that anything we set our minds to in the days before we die distracts our attention from death and thus offers some psychological value, but little more. And in some cases, no doubt that's true. However, it seemed plausible to me that many acts could have an impact that extends far beyond the individual. An intimate message, for instance, that touches friends and family. Or an ambitious novel that reaches much further.

More broadly, though, it seems to me that these last acts can also have an effect more globally, by shaping the way we think about human nature. Certainly, they're the stuff of myth and legend, and it's no surprise that they have such a prominent position in modern film and fiction. And just as these fictional last acts strike a chord in the public imagination, so, too, do real-life acts. For instance, the media's coverage of public disasters—the Sago mine explosion or the events of 9/11—gives last acts a prominent place. Long after many details of the 9/11 hijacking of United Flight 93 are forgotten, for instance, we'll still remember the passengers' efforts to crash the plane prematurely. So these acts are widely visible and, at least in some cases, become touchstones and defining elements of events.

And I wondered how these last acts shape our opinions of those who have died, and also of human nature more generally. How do these last acts provoke us to imagine what's possible? And how do they expand our ideas of what each of us is capable of? This is perhaps the most difficult set of questions that this book takes on, but ultimately, I think, the most rewarding.

Together, all of these questions became the inspiration for this book when I decided that they're answerable. That realization came on slowly and was prompted—forced, really—by repeated encounters with my patients that led me back to this topic again and again. But I realized, too, that these answers couldn't—and shouldn't—come only from my patients.

Meaningful, generalizable answers, I thought, would need to come from a wide range of examples. From history, for instance, and from biographies. And also from film and literature, even poetry. Nor could answers come solely from my experience as a physician. Instead, I'd need a variety of methods. Psychology, ethics, anthropology, neuropsychology, and even economics, I decided, would all have a contribution to make.

So this book draws on a wide range of sources and methods to understand how we respond when we're faced with death, and how we choose to spend the time that we have left. The answers are sometimes heartening, sometimes dismaying, and often both. In isolation, each person's response is a Rorschach blot that reaffirms whatever we know about an individual and whatever we believe about human nature. But taken together, and examined in an organized way, the themes that make up this part of the human experience are the bare structure of who we are, or at least who we'd like to be, if we had enough time.

Examples and Styles

It's all very well to describe a taxonomy of last acts, and interesting, I think, to understand why we make the choices that we do. And it will be helpful, too, if I can explain why I think that some last acts are better than others. But I suspect this book's real value to most readers will lie elsewhere.

For most of us, Sylvester's question is one that we will ask at some point. Most of us will die of chronic progressive illnesses like cancer, emphysema, dementia, or heart disease. And most of us, therefore, will have enough time to be able to make choices about how we want to spend whatever time we have left.

Sylvester's story serves as my own, nagging reminder of this. And his predicament is hardly unique. I'm certain that many of my patients are overwhelmed by the enormity of the task they've been given. How best to spend the days or weeks they have in front of them? It's a question that has considerable weight because of its significance both to them and to their families.

But it's also a perplexing question, because there are so many possible answers. How, then, to make the best choices—from among an infinite array—in the right way? This is a question that, ultimately, many of my patients feel they're not able to answer, or at least to answer well.

And if this is true of patients facing terminal illness whose time can be measured in months, and whose friends and family are close at hand, then it is certainly true of those who die unexpectedly in coal mine disasters, shipwrecks, and the like. Without warning, and without time to consider, it would be surprising indeed if people in those situations managed to make choices that were the best possible ones for them. Particularly when many people—coal miners, for instance—find themselves thrown together. Buffeted by the choices of others, it's difficult to imagine that anyone could hope to make one that is unique and genuinely their own.

More generally, most people faced with their own impending death lack the intellectual resources to make the best possible use of the time they have. I don't mean intelligence, unless perhaps you count emotional intelligence. It's just that very few of us, myself included, have the capacity to engage the question of what we should do with the unrestrained enthusiasm that the question requires of us.

But some do. And what really is most compelling, and what's driven me in writing this book, are those special examples—from among my patients and others—of last acts that are both unique and uniquely perfect. These are the stories that make up the backbone of this book, and they all describe people who took the measure of the frame in which they found themselves and made within it an individual statement.

Sometimes these are writers, or academics who have the time, resources, and emotional intelligence to reflect on their experiences. And sometimes these are other people—engineers, teachers, gardeners, and housewives—who are utterly unremarkable except for the way they manage to transform the last days of their lives. All of them, every single one, had a style, an imprint that was immediately recognizable.

And nowhere is that style so vibrant and flamboyant as it is in Anatole Broyard's account of his last year with prostate cancer. In fact, "style" was precisely the word that Broyard himself used. "I really think you have to have a style in which you finish your life" he wrote. "That's what I'm doing right now. I'm finishing my life."

His style, to use his term, was enthusiastic and almost joyous. What is so remarkable to me about Broyard's account is that he fully inhabited the last year of life that he was given. Even the metaphor he used fits: "At the end, you're posing for eternity. It's your last picture."

And Broyard devotes as much attention to exploring the borders and corners of that picture as he does to its center. Others faced with the same diagnosis would have concentrated their attention, perhaps, on their illness and impending death. But he saw his illness as new territory, full of discovery and opportunity. Even his relationship with his physician gave space to invent: ". . . when my doctor comes in, I juggle him. I toss him about. I throw him from hand to hand, and he hardly knows what to do with me. I never act sick. A puling person is not appealing." (To "pule," by the way—I didn't know what it meant either—is to whine or whimper.)

This enthusiasm and style has become, for me, emblematic of the way that all of us could inhabit our last days. It's not the specific gestures that are so inspiring, although I still smile every time I read Broyard's description of the way he manages his doctor. It is instead the intoxicating energy with which he chooses these gestures, matching and interweaving them to create the most beautiful picture he can imagine. He even wryly suggests a contest: "So I think we should have a competition in dying, sort of like Halloween costumes. I think you should try to die the most beautiful death you can. Let's give a prize for the most beautiful death. We can call it heaven."

Although Broyard enlisted his own sense of style to create a beautiful and coherent image of his last year of life, style is not defined solely by beauty. Indeed, others writers—several of whom were Broyard's contemporaries—composed their final pictures with a very different style. For instance, when Harold Brodkey wrote about his diagnosis of AIDS and the events that led up to his death, he did so with a truculence that was self-deprecating and genuinely funny. Rather than a beautiful death, he said, he wanted a death that would be interesting. "I wanted to have the most interesting illness, if not in my apartment house, then at least in my apartment," he wrote. "I was tired of being unimportant."

Ultimately, brief vignettes can't capture the style of either writer. But if Broyard's last days were painted, they would resemble a Jackson Pollock, perhaps, with exuberant colors and sinuous shapes flung together. Brodkey's, on the other hand, might be illustrated by the postmodern irony of an artist like Julian Schnabel. You could object to those characterizations—I recognize they're not a perfect fit—but you'd have to admit that Broyard and Brodkey each brought a sense of style to their last days, and that those styles were singularly their own.

The most important point, though, is that a sense of style gave Broyard, Brodkey, and others an organizing principle that protected them from being overwhelmed by endless possibilities, as Sylvester was. For someone with a developed sense of personal style, some choices are natural, while most are irrelevant. Brodkey, I think, was guided by a mulishly stubborn self-criticism tempered by love, just as Broyard could not really have spent his time in any other way than in an ebullient celebration of beauty.

Style for the Rest of Us

But what about the rest of us—and I count myself in this group—who don't have a sense of style to guide them? I would be no more likely to inhabit my last days with the style of Broyard or Brodkey than I would be to inhabit a park bench with the style that Cartier-Bresson's lady was able to achieve accidentally. Nor, I suspect, would most of us.

Simply borrowing one of those styles—say, Brodkey's irony and distance—would certainly not serve any of us well. Those styles would not have suited me any better that they would have suited Sylvester. And even though Brodkey's account resonated for me in a way that I didn't find with others, and offered a narrative that I thought I could place myself in, his style was uniquely his own. So these examples don't offer us off-the-shelf patterns for our last days.

What I'd hope for instead is a dialogue in which we can learn from the choices of those who have made them thoughtfully. That's what I've tried to create in these pages. And in assembling these stories, I've tried to call on people like Broyard, Brodkey, and a few dozen others, including many of my patients, whose choices and styles can help us to define our own.

I imagine, for instance, what Sylvester might have learned from three men who shared a single land line on the ninety-second floor of one of the World Trade Center towers in the Carr Futures conference room, placing calls to friends and families about ten minutes before the tower collapsed. What could those men have told Sylvester about what he could say, and what was important? What was really, truly important, after you strip away the clutter of our everyday conversations?

Perhaps someone like Broyard or Brodkey would have been able to grasp the essence of a message that Sylvester could have offered. Or perhaps they would have glimpsed the outline of an idea that Sylvester didn't know was there. Maybe they could have helped him to fill in that outline, creating a last image that would fit the frame of his circumstances.

Finally, maybe there is someone whose style and example Sylvester might have recognized and responded to. Because even though Broyard has his own sense of style that allowed him to inhabit his last days as naturally, and as perfectly, as a bespoke suit, he was also enthusiastically appreciative of the styles of others. "A hospital is full of wonderful and terrible stories" he wrote, "and if I were a doctor I would read them as one reads good fiction and let them educate me." And it's really the potentialities of these imagined juxtapositions, and the resultant exchanges that they might inspire and provoke, that have made writing this book so enjoyable for me.

Sylvester

Sylvester could sense the opportunity he faced. In fact, he recognized it before I did. He understood that he could make of that opportunity whatever he wanted and, I think, was overwhelmed by that opportunity, and by the endless choices that he could make. In a sense, I think, he was frozen by the enormity of the task in front of him.

How could he possibly fill the time he had left in a way that is commensurate with the magnitude of the opportunity? What words and gestures would be significant enough—and would carry enough weight—to justify his time? It would be tragic not to fully use the time he had, but doubly tragic, perhaps, to exhaust that time on words and gestures that were trivial.

This portrayal of Sylvester's state of mind is speculative but not, I think, too far wrong. After he left the hospital to go home with hospice care, he would ask his question of the hospice nurse and later his daughter, who then asked me. I wish I could say that I was able to offer an answer the second time, but I wasn't.

So his question was clearly important to him, and perhaps even a bit of an obsession. It may also have been a question to which he had given some thought before his diagnosis. Indeed, he had suspected long before his dull-witted physician did that he had cancer and would have had ample time to imagine the question and to become convinced of its significance. Though not enough time, apparently, to formulate an answer.

Still, despite the intensity with which Sylvester seemed to focus on the question of how he should spend his time, his last days were much like those of my other patients. He lived for about five weeks after our conversation that night in his hospital room, and in that time he made a few choices. Some were important, and many were necessary, but most were trivial. He went home, which was what he wanted. He reviewed his will, although as far as I know he didn't make any changes. He saw a few friends from his neighborhood and of course he saw his family. But for the most part, he waited to die.

Perhaps his final days were so ordinary precisely because of the intensity with which he'd tried to decide how to use those days. There were, really, far too many choices. I imagine that, for Sylvester and indeed for many of us, facing these choices for the first time must be a bit like walking into an enormous clothing store without the guidance that a clear idea of one's own style might provide. He probably felt overwhelmed by countless options, and yet he seemed to know that any choice would be both enormously significant and irrevocably final.

All in all, the last month or so of Sylvester's life was not a work of art. The way he used his time was, ultimately, the same way that most of my patients use their time—an admixture of daily activities and obligations, interspersed occasionally with a few notable events. I'm left to conclude that he didn't live his last days in the way that he thought he had an obligation to live them.

But he could have. He was ready, like the mason he'd once been, to get to work. Or almost ready, because there was something else he seemed to need: examples and options. The stones that he could fit in place.

And so that's ultimately what this book is. It's a collection of examples and stories that I wish I could have shared with Sylvester that night. As I wrote this book, trying to capture the style that propels each one, I imagined Sylvester weighing them one at a time, judging its contours and weight, and perhaps finding the one that would have been the perfect fit.

ONE

Jacob

Fighting and Survival

Jacob

Throughout the long, tumultuous night that I took care of him, Jacob knew he wouldn't survive to leave the hospital, yet he stead-fastly refused to act as if he were dying. And as his death grew closer, those of us who were huddled around his bed became in-creasingly insistent, and strident, in imploring him to plan for the end that we all knew was coming and to make the best possible use of the time he had left. But the proximity to death that heightened our sense of urgency seemed only to solidify Jacob's resolve to keep on fighting.

Before Jacob became my patient that night, he'd been a graduate student in film at the University of Iowa and had lived on the edge of town in a large apartment that was lined with classic film posters. He had a fiancée, Marylee, and a large extended family living nearby. He had a vintage Norton Model 2 motorcycle from 1925 that he had rebuilt in his living room, over Marylee's sullen objections. And he had a particularly aggressive form of leukemia that was almost universally fatal.

By the time I met him, Jacob had been through countless rounds of chemotherapy and a "salvage" bone marrow transplant, which was a last attempt to cure his leukemia after it had recurred. All of these treatments came with horrendous complications and discomfort but had helped Jacob to live five years since his diagnosis. On average, only 5 percent of patients with the same kind of leukemia live that long, a statistic that put Jacob at the head of his class. Still, he hadn't yet reached the cure that he and Marylee had hoped for.

At a clinic visit about a week earlier, Jacob's oncologist had found a mild pancytopenia—a lowered blood-cell count across all cell types—that worried him. Those low cell counts might have been the aftershocks of Jacob's last round of chemotherapy, or they might have been due to a vitamin deficiency, drug toxicity, or any one of a number of relatively benign causes. Or they might have been the first sign that his leukemia had relapsed. But Jacob didn't want to have a bone marrow biopsy done at that visit and had planned to come back the following week. Like his oncologist, Jacob had been worried, but he wasn't really anxious. He'd endured enough ambiguous test results over the years not to be overly concerned.

A few days later, the last Friday in July, Jacob felt more tired than usual. So he called in sick at his job as a teaching assistant and spent the morning in bed with a fever, sleeping and watching television. A brief phone call that morning stoked his oncologist's concerns. What worried him the most—enough to make a last-minute appointment for Jacob—was the absence of any upper respiratory symptoms that might have indicated a benign cause for his symptoms, like a simple viral illness. But by midafternoon, Jacob felt better, and he called to cancel his appointment and went back to sleep.

When Marylee returned to their apartment that evening, Jacob was confused and half-asleep, unsure of where he was. And he also had shaking chills and shortness of breath that concerned her enough to pile him into her car and drive straight to the hospital. She was worried, but calmly efficient, since she had been through this sort of thing before. Late nights in the emergency room were as commonplace for the two of them as more traditional nights out at the bars near campus were for other couples. She knew the ER nurses by name, which was a comfort. Less reassuring, though, were memories of the nail-biting waits that the two of them had endured while lab tests determined whether the latest problem was a minor incident or a major event.

Still, for Marylee, this late-night trip across town was one of many. More frustrating, probably, since she knew that Jacob should have kept his appointment that afternoon. But Jacob had lived through many late-night trips to the ER, and if there were warning flags flying, Marylee hadn't seen them.

Those flags were flying, though. And they quickly became visible to everyone on duty in the ER, and especially to Lisa, who was the charge nurse that night. She went out into the ambulance drop zone as soon as she recognized Marylee's old white Subaru wagon with a prominent "FARMS NOT ARMS" bumper sticker covering half the rusted tailgate. She saw immediately that Jacob was very short of breath and that he was unstable enough, she thought, to be put in the trauma room where he could be put on a ventilator quickly if he became unable to breathe on his own. Lisa and Marylee conferred in the windy hangarlike vestibule, bracketed by two pairs of sliding glass doors that separated the ambulance drop zone from the ER, as the staff hurried Jacob inside. And a few minutes later Jacob lay in the trauma room, surrounded by an array of devices—IV pumps, a ventilator, a defibrillator—that offered a crude foreshadowing of how Jacob's life was likely to end.

I was already in the ER that night, part of an informal tribunal that would decide whether another patient should go to me or to the cardiac ICU, and so I overheard some of the conversations between Lisa and the ER attending, who waved me over. He was an oddly formal physician. Not old, but with proper old-school mannerisms he had picked up from the local general practitioners he had worked for while growing up in a small rural town. And as a general practitioner might have, he told me about Jacob's medical history, and about his family, and about Marylee. It was more detail than I needed, and certainly more than I would have gleaned from any other ER physician, but it was welcome context nonetheless. And—in a ceremonial gesture that, sadly, has gone the way of house calls—he escorted me across the ER to the trauma room to introduce me to Jacob in person.

My first impression of Jacob from the door of the trauma room, as we stood 8 or 10 feet away, was that he looked surprisingly vigorous. It's true that his skin seemed washed out and depleted. But that was mostly the result of the ER's unflattering fluorescent lights, whose effects were, at least, rigidly democratic, forcing a pallor of chronic illness on both doctors and patients alike.

Despite that, Jacob didn't look at all like someone with a chronic, serious illness. He had the solid, meaty look of a wrestler, and bristle-stiff rust-colored hair that was brushed back in a tight helmet. And across his face and upper chest above the hospital gown I could see a wide expanse of freckles that were, I later learned, the result of summer afternoons spent on sailboats at the University of Iowa's "Yacht Club" on Lake McBride. He certainly didn't look like someone who found himself once again standing on death's doorstep, waiting to see whether this would be the time that he would be ushered inside.

Yet as the attending and I watched Jacob from the doorway, we needed only a few seconds to see that his respiratory rate, about 40 breaths/minute, was dangerously high. A normal rate is about 15 breaths/minute, and one as high as Jacob's was worrisome because most people can't sustain that level of effort for long. When he could no longer breathe rapidly enough to get the oxygen that he needed and to blow off carbon dioxide, I knew that we would need to sedate him and place him on a mechanical ventilator.

I was thinking about all of this, and making a note to myself to call the respiratory technician to let her know to get a ventilator ready, when I realized that Jacob had shifted his head slightly to the side and was looking at us. But intermittently. He would look toward us for one or two coarse, raspy breaths, and then back at the ceiling, as if we were an unwanted distraction. Or perhaps, I thought later that night, as if his energy and attention were consumed by the effort of breathing and he couldn't spare more than a glance for us.

Introductions were brief. Jacob couldn't force words in between rapid, urgent breaths, and instead simply offered a handshake that was sweaty and awkward but surprisingly tenacious. Taking turns, the attending and I sketched the barest outlines of his situation. Perhaps, we said, his symptoms were the result of aggressive pneumonia, which we could probably treat. Or perhaps they were due to a fulminant recurrence of his leukemia, which we couldn't. We told him, too, about what would happen over the next few hours. He would be taken to the ICU, where we would do an emergency bronchoscopy—a look into his lungs with a small, flexible, optical device—to try to reach a quick diagnosis. And we'd also be talking with him about the sorts of treatments he would and wouldn't want.

Throughout our abbreviated explanation, which didn't take more than a few minutes, Jacob stared fixedly at the ceiling. He would glance at us occasionally, but would only meet our gaze if we stood over him, in his field of vision. He didn't say anything, but would squeeze my hand intermittently in response to some of the most important points.

A few minutes later, as I disengaged my hand from his to make preparations for moving him, I realized that, without the structure of eye contact or any verbal exchange, I had been filling in my own interpretation of his hand's pressure as understanding, acknowledgment, and tacit consent. Back at the door to the trauma room, talking with Lisa, I looked back at Jacob, who was still breathing far too rapidly, his eyes locked on the ceiling. And I considered for a moment that maybe Jacob hadn't heard anything we had said.

It was after midnight when Lisa and I wheeled Jacob's gurney headfirst down the hospital's silent grey-carpeted hallways, with Marylee tucked in behind us like an honor guard. Jacob didn't speak as we left the ER through the rear entrance, husbanding his strength for each breath. His eyes were rolled upward, anticipating our direction and registering each overhead fluorescent panel with a rapid downward tic.

I plotted a route that bypassed the usual service elevators in the back of the building and instead nudged the gurney toward the public elevators in the hospital lobby. That detour was partly to save time. Mostly, though, I wanted to make sure that the code team could find us quickly with a crash cart if Jacob had a respiratory arrest on the way. But he didn't, and we arrived in the ICU to find several nurses and the respiratory technician waiting for us. Their extra efficiency, and the apprehensiveness it concealed, made me realize that I was surprised we'd made it.

Saturday mornings in the ICU were typically calm. Admissions from the night before had been tucked in, new problems either hadn't developed or hadn't been recognized, and the next admissions were still a few hours away. The muted beeping of alarms and the rhythmic breathing of the mechanical ventilators next to most of the beds created a sort of white noise that softened the normal tensions of the unit's life-and-death struggles. But Jacob's corner bed was soon fluttering with activity that was amplified by Marylee's incursions, whenever the nursing staff let her in.

In his first hour on the unit, we gave Jacob a wide range of treatments—everything we could think of, in fact—to try to improve his breathing. We used 100 percent oxygen, for instance, and inhaled medications to open airway passages, and steroids given intravenously. Finally, during a tense hour in which we were ready to put him on a ventilator, Jacob's breathing became a little easier, at least to the point at which he could speak in partial sentences. Still, we knew that what we were seeing was no more than a temporary reprieve. Steve, the ICU attending, did a quick and anxious bronchoscopy that showed what Jacob's oncologist had been afraid of: lungs infiltrated by leukemic cells that stained a deep and dangerous purple under the microscope.

I had a covert conference with Steve and Alicia, Jacob's nurse, at the nursing station at the other end of the unit. We spoke furtively, our heads down over another patient's chart, knowing that any indication that we were discussing Jacob would draw Marylee toward us. Mercifully, his extended family hadn't arrived yet. But they were thirty minutes away at most, so we didn't have much time. We weren't avoiding them, but we needed some time to think things through.

None of us wanted to put Jacob on a ventilator. That much we could agree on easily. Doing so would require heavy sedation, taking away his last few hours of consciousness that he might use to say goodbye to his family. Nor could we see any benefit of using a ventilator, because Jacob had very little time left no matter what we did. Without a ventilator, he'd die in the next few hours. With a ventilator, he might survive the night, but we were sure he'd die the following day. The leukemia in his lungs was so pervasive that chemotherapy wouldn't help him and even steroids, which are often useful in some types of leukemia, wouldn't buy him any time.

Instead, we thought the best approach would be to treat Jacob's shortness of breath as aggressively as we could. In addition to oxygen, we'd use morphine to decrease the sensation of breathlessness and lorazepam, an antianxiety drug, to help him to relax. And there were other strategies—tricks, really—that we planned to use, like positioning Jacob so that his respiratory muscles could work more efficiently, and placing a fan by the bedside.

We were certain that all of these interventions could make Jacob more comfortable, and we tried to convey our sense of confidence by telling him about each one. We described what we could do for him in detail—almost certainly in more detail than Jacob wanted—in a clamorous effort to prove to him that we wouldn't relax our own efforts to make him comfortable. Finally, we promised him that if we weren't able to control his shortness of breath through other means, we could give him a sedative medication that would induce a light sleep. This was the alternative to a ventilator that we offered, and it was one that we thought was truly the better option.

But it became clear that a ventilator was exactly what Jacob wanted. More generally, he wanted us to do everything we could to keep him alive as long as possible, even treatment that would only buy him a few hours during which he would be unconscious. Jacob told us unambiguously, and repeatedly, that he wanted to die receiving all the treatment we could offer, and we could say nothing, it seemed, that would soften his resolve.

Those conversations, if you could call them that, were among the most difficult that any of us had ever had. With each breath he tensed his neck and shoulders and pushed down on the bed with both hands, as if that might open a little more air space in lungs that were densely lined with leukemia cells. His exhalations came in painful gasps—little more than grunts—that inserted jagged spaces into his normally fluid speech. Yet despite the warning of death's proximity that came with each breath, Jacob continued to insist that he wanted every additional minute of life that we could offer him.

And those conversations were particularly difficult for Alicia. Like Steve and I, she knew that Jacob was going to die that night. In addition, though, she was engaged to be married to an orthopedics resident that fall. That gave her a unique view of Jacob's choice to pursue all possible treatment and she became increasingly angry and eventually tearful when she realized what Jacob wanted. Alicia couldn't believe that Jacob would let go, or "throw away" (her phrase) Marylee and his family, prematurely. She saw more clearly than I did that every minute that Jacob spent arguing with us, or inhaling yet another breathing treatment, was a minute that he wasn't able to spend with them.

Prognosis and Uncertainty

Jacob's story shows as clearly as that of any other patient I've ever taken care of just how strong the magnetism of hope and survival can be. Keep in mind that Jacob wasn't making decisions about cancer treatment that offered a small increase in survival in exchange for some discomfort and inconvenience. His was an all-or-nothing choice to give up a last chance for meaningful interaction with family in exchange for a few hours of a heavily-sedated facsimile of life.

Jacob's leukemia was highly unusual—a medical curiosity that affects fewer than 1,000 people every year. Yet his situation and the choices that he made are not at all unique. Every year in the United States alone, over 300,000 patients die in intensive care units, and many of these die receiving treatments that offer no meaningful chance of benefit. Indeed, this path to death is so well traveled that it often seems as if the primary way—and perhaps the only way—that people choose to spend their last hours of life is by struggling against overwhelming odds. When faced with a choice of how to spend one's final moments, in fact, the dominant response may be to reject that premise entirely and seek instead to change the rules of the game, buying a few more days.

Perhaps we should assume that when someone like Jacob is faced with what amounts to a death sentence, there is usually enough doubt, hope, and faith to make survival a possibility. Not a good possibility, and in numeric terms perhaps not even a measurable one. But for most people, in most situations, a possibility of survival has enough influence to perturb and rearrange other priorities.

This influence may not always be visible. Indeed, it has become masked, lately, by the increasingly prominent concept of "a good death." Although each of us is likely to have his or her own idea of what a good death would be, interviews with varied populations of patients and health care providers have elicited attributes that have proven to be remarkably homogeneous. Common themes to emerge from these studies, for instance, include freedom from excessive suffering, peace, a sense of dignity, and connection with friends and family.

The idea of a good death is a compelling one, especially when viewed from a distance by people in good health. But that idea may not actually motivate decisions until very late in the course of illness. Indeed, some have found an emphasis on peaceful, dignified dying to be oppressive if it is introduced too soon. Stephen Jay Gould wrote with some humor and more than a bit of anger about his own encounter with a rare form of cancer and his decision to fight despite the bleak prognosis that he was given. In doing so he defended his decision in a popular science article, and mounted a preemptive counterattack, complete with a nod to Dylan Thomas, on the notion of a good death:

> *It has become, in my view, a bit too trendy to regard the acceptance of death as something tantamount to intrinsic dignity. Of course I agree with the preacher of Ecclesiastes that there is a time to live and a time to die—and when my skein runs out I hope to face the end calmly and in my own way. For most situations, however, I prefer the more martial view that death is the ultimate enemy—and I find nothing reproachable in those who rage mightily against the dying of the light.*

Gould's dry humor disguises the strength of his feelings, feelings that are readily apparent elsewhere in the article as he argues persuasively that median survival figures tell patients and their physicians very little that is clinically useful. Particularly seen within the frame of his own initially successful fight against cancer, Gould's argument appears incontestable. And this is the real hegemony that a desire for survival has over us. For Gould, and in fact for most of us, a hope of survival is so powerful, and so enveloping, that it's surprising that any of us will choose to use our time in other ways.

Health Care Decisions Near the End of Life

To understand the force that a desire for survival exerts even in the last hours and minutes of life, it's useful to turn first to studies of decision-making in health care settings. Of course, the circumstances of dying in a hospital are very different than those of a plane crash, a mining accident, or a natural disaster. Still, studies of decision-making near the end of life typically involve people—patients—who know that they have a serious illness. And they know, too, that they're likely to die very soon. So these are studies of people whose choices about life and death are made with adequate information.

If this seems like a trivial point, consider the array of other situations in which people die and how little information many of them have about their chances of survival. For instance, when nineteen miners were trapped after an explosion in the Springhill, Nova Scotia, mining disaster of 1958, the mood of the group alternated initially between resignation and wild hope. On the first day, the miners expected a rescue at any moment. They would become wildly elated at the sound of falling rocks, interpreting them as the signs of an approaching rescue team even though at that point the extent of the collapse was not yet known and missing miners had not even been identified. Over the next several days, the miners' hopes began to wane as their meager food supply—crusts of sandwiches and apple cores leftover from their lunch break—disappeared. But it was then that rescue teams were working eighteen-hour shifts only a few hundred feet away.

In contrast, most people who die in a health care setting will have enough information to allow a prediction of death with a reasonable degree of confidence. For Jacob, certainly, we felt that we could predict his death with absolute certainty. And all of this information creates a laboratory of sorts in which we can learn about how a hope of survival influences the choices that people make. And by understanding how that hope of survival operates in health care settings, we can gain a better appreciation for the pull that it has on people in other settings, where that information is limited or nonexistent.

Hope

Elisabeth Kübler-Ross's 1969 book *On Death and Dying* is generally credited with introducing the words "death" and "dying" into mainstream discourse. Indeed, it's these words by which her book is best remembered, which is ironic given that it is really about our tenacious grip on life and the reluctance with which most of us let go. At the heart of Kübler-Ross's book is the suggestion, based on interviews and her own experiences with her patients, that people faced with a terminal illness pass through recognizable "stages," from denial, through bargaining, to acceptance.

On Death and Dying was embraced widely and unquestioningly by many, but time and more extensive research have prompted critical scrutiny of the stages that Kübler-Ross proposed. These stages, it turns out, do not fit all patients, or perhaps even the majority. In fact, she admitted as much when she acknowledged that "even the most accepting, the most realistic patients left the possibility open for some cure." She goes on to describe the subtle way that hope of a cure "sneaks in" at unpredictable moments, offering a respite of denial that my patients rely on to endure what are all too often lonely and terrifying nights.

And this hope of a cure appears capriciously to disrupt the smooth progression from denial to acceptance that Kübler-Ross describes so pristinely. Throughout the course of an illness, hope wages a guerilla war and wreaks havoc on neat plans to taper treatments and limit aggressive therapy. Indeed, hope has become a major—arguably *the* major—theme of modern medicine.

Often the chance of survival is so small as to appear negligible. Nevertheless, that small chance exerts a disproportionate effect on the health care decisions that patients make. And because they've been so thoroughly studied, we know a great deal about the choices that patients make, or say that they would make, when the chance of survival is vanishingly small.

The Will to Live

We know, for instance, that about one in five Americans dies in an intensive care unit. We know, too, that among those who die in a hospital their odds of dying in an ICU are about one in two. These dying patients often receive all the treatment we can offer, including antibiotics, mechanical ventilation, dialysis, intravenous medications to maintain blood pressure, and a tangled web of tubes to monitor heart function, measure urine output, and provide nutrition. We also know that these experiences can be extraordinarily uncomfortable. Patients who survive, even if they are grateful to be alive, recall their ICU stay as something not too different from torture, marked by pain, shortness of breath, confusion, and often straps that restrain their arms and legs.

There is also strong evidence that many patients receive aggressive treatment because this is what they want. Terri Fried, a friend and researcher at Yale University, interviewed a group of patients who were seriously ill and had a limited life expectancy even with the most aggressive treatment. By using a series of "trade-off" questions, she was able to define the threshold at which each patient was willing to give up aggressive treatment. She found that the vast majority of these seriously ill patients said that they would accept the most aggressive possible treatment if doing so might return them to their current state of health.

And these preferences take shape in a wide range of clinical situations. In fact, some of the most surprising data about choices come from the decisions that patients with advanced cancer make when they decide to enroll in experimental Phase I trials. These are the first studies in which a potential cancer drug is tested in humans. These studies are designed to establish the drug's maximum tolerated dose, not to test its effectiveness. Patients are generally told that there is no chance of benefit for them and that the main reason to enroll in such a trial is to help future patients. Still, many patients do enroll in Phase I trials in hopes of an improved chance of survival, or perhaps even a cure. For instance, in one small study, Christopher Daugherty, an oncologist, found that 85 percent of patients in such trials said they were enrolling because of a hope of benefit to themselves.

The hope of survival is so powerful, in fact, that it can be mulishly unyielding in the face of reality. In a study that I did with several colleagues, we wanted to try to help patients to make decisions that were more realistic, given their prognosis and treatment options. A year into the study, though, we realized that our attempts to educate and inform patients were having virtually no effect. In fact, the conversations we had with patients often seemed to strengthen their resolve to pursue every possible treatment, which was hardly our intent. Admitting defeat, we revised the study and focused instead on helping those patients with more realistic preferences to talk to their physicians about their goals.

Explaining the Pursuit of Survival in the Face of Death

What was really inexplicable to those of us who took care of Jacob that night is that we knew he wouldn't survive for more than a day. And that knowledge made his desire for treatment qualitatively different from that of other patients we had cared for, and indeed it was fundamentally different from the circumstances of most studies of patients' choices. Even in Phase I oncology trials, successes do occur. Although the most ardent optimist would be forced to admit that the chance of remission in a Phase I trial is less than 1 percent, even the most incredulous pessimist would grant that it is greater than zero.

In contrast, we were certain—absolutely certain—that Jacob would never leave the hospital. And that certainty made his choice to pursue all possible treatment seem like an anomaly. It was, I thought, some sort of malfunction that would remain inexplicable. But several years later I happened across an example, from circumstances that could not have been more different, that made me realize that Jacob's choice that night was not the random event that I had assumed.

When the merchant brig *Commerce* ran aground on the west coast of Africa in 1815, Captain James Riley's order to abandon ship saved the crew but left them all stranded on the edge of the Sahara desert, hundreds of miles from the nearest settlement. After a series of bad choices and worse luck, the crew found themselves a week later severely dehydrated, without a boat, provisions, or water. In a vividly detailed history of the *Commerce*'s wreck, Dean King describes the crew's desperate efforts to climb the steep cliff that rose above the beach, and their utter hopelessness when they found nothing but endless desert. " 'Tis enough," King describes one of the crew as saying, "Here we must breathe our last."

There was, truly, no hope for the crew. Their situation was as hopeless, I thought, as Jacob's had been. Their best course was simply to lie down and to prepare to die. In fact, this was the feeling of many in the crew, and perhaps the majority.

Yet they continued, just as Jacob had. They began to walk, slowly and painfully, in a direction chosen more or less at random. Surrounded by a perfectly flat, empty and hostile desert, they suffered sharp stones that punctured their feet, as well as unbearable thirst and relentless sun that had left their exposed skin sloughing in painful sheets.

As I reread King's account, searching for a clue to what drove those men across the desert, I couldn't help remembering the eerily similar search that Steve and Alicia and I had pursued a few years before. And as I speculated about why the *Commerce* crew persevered I wondered, too, what it was that had driven Jacob that night. On the surface both stories seem to be about people who carry on in the face of overwhelming odds, hoping for a chance of rescue long after most people would have given up. But if it was plain that there was no real hope of survival—none at all—then both the *Commerce* crew and Jacob must have been motivated by other reasons. What might those reasons have been?

Regret Bias

Imagine that you're in Jacob's position and you believe that you won't survive to leave the hospital. In fact, you believe you probably won't live through the night. Although you suspect that there is an infinitesimal chance that you could, you don't think that possibility is worth considering, and you dismiss it. Instead, you decide to focus on other ways to use the few hours you have left, like spending time with family members who are with you, or writing a hasty note to those who aren't.

But as soon as you do, you start having second thoughts. Second thoughts and needling, harrying questions that demand that you reconsider. And while they're subtle at first, they gradually become more insistent.

What if a high dose of chemotherapy might buy me a few days? Or maybe there's an experimental protocol I'd be eligible for? Maybe . . . ?

Even if you firmly dismiss each of these questions—and Jacob certainly knew enough to try to push them from his mind—their persistence would gradually wear you down. The result would be an almost obsessive focus on these sorts of "What if?" scenarios, which are an all-consuming distraction that drains patients of energy.

In fact, throughout our lives, and in a wide variety of circumstances, we all make decisions that are designed to minimize the possibility of regret in the future. Some psychologists call this "regret bias," because they believe that the resulting choices are irrational, or "biased." But David Bell, Graham Loomes, and Robert Sugden, the first researchers to study this phenomenon in an organized way, found that people's choices are often more rational than they appear to be. That is, a person who chooses the less desirable of two options may appear to be making an irrational decision. But that decision begins to make sense if the person believes that the option he or she chose would be less likely to cause feelings of regret if it turned out to be the wrong choice.

I think that some form of regret bias influences many of the health care choices that my patients make, although probably not Jacob's, whose future was of course limited to a matter of hours. Still, it's possible that his choice had a related purpose. Perhaps, instead, he continued to pursue treatment in order to silence the insistent voice of anxiety that would have told him that there was something else he could be doing. That a ventilator or steroids, or some other treatment, just might buy him a little more time. The easiest way for him to silence that voice would have been to make the decision that it was urging. He would try any treatment that was available. And perhaps that choice gave him a sort of peace in knowing—absolutely and without question—that he was doing everything that he could.

In retrospect, I think it's possible that something like this was playing out in Jacob's mind that night. He didn't share it with us, and perhaps he couldn't. And I'm almost certain that he didn't share it with Marylee or his family. But I think these nagging thoughts might have played a role in his choices, leading him down a path of aggressive treatment that was not going to prolong his life but which may at least have quieted his anxiety and his fears of regret.

Routines and Habits

It's possible, too, that Jacob's choice of aggressive treatment was simply the easiest one for him to make that night. Not physically easier, of course, but cognitively easier. Many of my patients who live for years with a serious illness, as Jacob did, seem to develop elaborate routines of treatment and self-assessment that provide structure and a sort of directional guidance. And they also develop relationships associated with those routines. Over time, all of these routines and relationships seem to wear grooves that resist a change in direction. So perhaps it was easier for Jacob to continue to pursue the same course than it was to stop, regroup, and consider other priorities and goals in the time he had left.

I think this phenomenon, or something like it, might partially explain Jacob's requests for aggressive treatment. He was used to thinking in terms of survival, and he was accustomed to measuring his course, often from hour to hour, by lab tests that pointed to interventions. Moreover, from what others have told me, this had always seemed to be the sole focus of his interactions with Marylee and, to a lesser extent, with his family.

So although Jacob could have refused a ventilator and turned instead to making the most of the time he had left, doing so would have deeply rearranged the plot of his interactions with his family and particularly with Marylee. Conversations that used to have a predicable content and cadence would suddenly have been blank and unprogrammed. Jacob, his family, and Marylee would have had to create a new vocabulary—very quickly—in a process that was bound to be uncomfortable. Perhaps, to Jacob, that discomfort was more daunting than the alternative of continued, if futile, treatment.

When I say that Jacob may have shied away from these sorts of last-hour conversations, I don't mean to imply that he was impassive, or apathetic. From what I know, and from what I heard from others, he was warm and generous and had an openness tempered by a dry sense of humor that gave him a large circle of close friends. So I could envision him spending his last night with friends and family, saying goodbye and even celebrating. In fact, it's the naturalness of that scene that makes Jacob's decision to die isolated on a ventilator so difficult for me to understand, and so tragic.

The Expectations of Others

Although it's possible that Jacob's choice that night was his way of stifling anxious regrets, or guarding comfortable patterns, these explanations seem to me to be incomplete. The problem, I think, is that they focus exclusively on Jacob and his state of mind. But patients like Jacob with chronic serious illnesses live in, and are supported by, a dense and seemingly infinite web of relationships and expectations. So even though explanations that focus on Jacob himself tend to be more salient, they ignore everyone else—friends, family, health care providers—who were with Jacob that night, and in the weeks and months before he died.

That the influence of others can have a pervasive effect on patients' choices was a lesson I learned early, when I was still doing a fellowship in palliative medicine at the University of Pennsylvania. A fellow inhabits a level in the medical hierarchy in between that of an attending physician and a resident. So my indeterminate place in the medical pecking order was often awkward, and I was careful to avoid causing offense and derailing the palliative care consult service that my mentor, Dr. Janet Abrahm, had worked so hard to build. Still, this very awkwardness was occasionally providential when patients turned to me to communicate with their physicians by passing loosely coded messages.

Janet once asked me to see an older man with multiple myeloma, a type of cancer that involves white blood cells. Lawrence was in his seventies but had an Aruba tan and tennis club body that had kept him looking at least twenty years younger. And from the door of his private room Lawrence looked exactly like what he was, the retired CEO of a successful manufacturing company.

But that doorway image was misleading. Over the past nine months or so his cancer had crept into virtually all of his bones, crowding out the normal cells and causing intense, unremitting pain. When I took a few steps into the room, his pallor and clenched jaw told the real story.

He was brusque, and almost rude, when I first met him. And my clumsy efforts to engage him in a discussion of his goals for treatment elicited curt responses or an angry silence. He wanted all possible treatment. Everything—whatever it takes. That was all he'd say.

Whether his abrupt replies were the result of his pain, my status, my inept questions, or just his managerial style, I couldn't tell. In any event, our first job was to manage his pain, and we did that with a combination of anti-inflammatory drugs, steroids, and opioids. Within a few hours he was resting comfortably, by later that evening he was smiling, and by the next day he was charming the nurses—a good sign.

It was on a quick follow-up visit the following afternoon that he invited me to sit on the edge of his bed. He looked uncomfortable, almost embarrassed, which put me on my guard. I began to envision some sort of deathbed confession of corporate malfeasance, marital duplicity, or worse.

In fact, he wanted to know whether the treatments he was getting were really keeping his multiple myeloma contained. He didn't think the treatments were doing any good, and, in truth, he was probably right. He asked me to confirm his suspicions and I did, but only reluctantly, and very delicately.

I didn't want to get caught, like a double agent, in between Lawrence and his physician. But I also thought he should know the truth, which was that his elaborate treatment regimen probably wouldn't slow his cancer's spread. And that was more or less what I told him.

In an instant his expression was rearranged. For a moment I thought I saw something like a gleam of hopefulness. But I saw a firm resolve, too, as if the successful executive had finally heard the suggestion that he'd been waiting for. So I'd recommend stopping his treatment, he wanted to know?

Well . . . it wasn't that simple. . . . And I couldn't say for sure. He should ask his oncologist.

Until that point our conversation had fallen into an easy banter, and Lawrence had even laughed with what I thought was a healthy cynicism about the treatment he'd been receiving. But at my suggestion that he talk to his oncologist, he looked down and began picking at his bedclothes, twisting two corners of his hospital sheet—tightly, in opposite directions—around his index fingers. He was suddenly even more apprehensive than he had been at the start of our conversation.

He had hoped that I would ask his oncologist for him, he said nervously. And after some prodding, he admitted that he didn't want to "disappoint" his oncologist, who had walked beside him every step of the long path that had led him here from his diagnosis, over five years ago. Throughout that time they had become close, and his oncologist had even attended Lawrence's granddaughter's wedding. Perhaps more significantly, his oncologist had also helped Lawrence through several difficult patches, including a hospitalization for pneumonia three months earlier that could easily have ended his life. So Lawrence's insistence on aggressive treatment was a front that was mostly, if not entirely, for his oncologist's benefit.

In a twist that would be worthy of an O. Henry story, Janet and I knew that his oncologist didn't want to continue Lawrence's treatment either. He had confessed as much to Janet first, and later to me. I was dismayed, but she was dismissive. "We see this all the time," she said, implying that once I gained a little experience, I would, too. "It's a little like hearing confession," she explained. "Patients often tell us what they don't want to tell their primary physicians."

The result in Lawrence's case was a treatment regimen that even he realized didn't make much sense. Why? Because Lawrence thought he was doing what his oncologist would want and his oncologist was doing what he thought Lawrence would want. So his curt demand that we do "whatever it takes" wasn't as simple as it had seemed. What appeared to be a steadfast insistence on receiving the most aggressive possible treatment was in fact a story of a relationship, expectations, and poor communication.

Janet and I met his oncologist in the elevator later that day and summarized Lawrence's concern about his treatment and his anxiety about being a disappointment. The oncologist was philosophical about stopping chemotherapy, saying that it had been worth a try, but that he didn't really believe it had done much good. And he wasn't at all troubled to hear that his patient had accepted the chemotherapy regimen with enthusiasm, even gratitude, because he thought that was what his oncologist expected. Like Janet, he had heard this before.

I later learned from his oncologist that once Lawrence had the opportunity to discuss his treatment options, he started to reassume his own confident managerial style. In particular, he became more assertive about reducing his treatment and refusing tests that had become routine. He enrolled in hospice a month after I met him, managing the nurses and home health aides like an executive marshaling his employees, and died at home about three months later.

I think Lawrence's motivation is a common one, and probably far more common that most of us physicians want to admit. It has occurred to me many times that Jacob could have been motivated by a fear of disappointing his physician. But I'm not sure. Jacob's oncologist was always frankly—some would say brutally—honest with his patients. Certainly, the rest of us in the ICU that night made our recommendations as plainly as we could. At least I hope we did. So I still think that Jacob's motivation, if it were anything other than a true wish to live as long as possible, was something else.

A Final Battle

I'd almost forgotten about Jacob a few years later when I got a holiday card from Lisa, the ER charge nurse who helped me admit him that night. Her card reached me at the hospital, and I opened it on the train on the way home that night. Thinking about my time in Iowa and the patients I had taken care of there brought me to Jacob, and back to the question of his motivation.

I looked out through the hazy Plexiglas of the commuter train as we rumbled by an old theater that played classics, and I noticed that this week there was a John Wayne special that ended, fittingly, with *The Shootist*, the last film Wayne ever made. It was an unsettling juxtaposition and an improbable coincidence. I felt like I was following a somewhat contrived film plot myself.

The story line of *The Shootist* revolves around an aging John Bernard Books (Wayne), who learns that he has cancer that will kill him. His physician (Jimmy Stewart) describes the horrors of a death from cancer and tells him, "You're a brave man. If I was a brave man, I wouldn't die like that." So Brooks decides to "go down fighting" rather than let cancer destroy him piece by piece. He says goodbye to Bond Rogers (Lauren Bacall) and, in director Don Siegel's predictable style, takes a gang of bad guys with him. (There is a common belief that Wayne himself was dying of stomach cancer while *The Shootist* was being filmed. To the best of my knowledge, that's not true. Still, by all accounts Wayne was in poor health during the filming. He had had surgery for lung cancer in 1964 and would in fact die of stomach cancer in 1979, only three years after the movie came out. Moreover, Lauren Bacall's husband Humphrey Bogart had died of esophageal cancer in 1956. So although it would be unwise to overstate parallels between real life and fiction, it's safe to say that for the key players, Wayne and Bacall, there was probably a personal meaning in the film's story.)

I began to wonder, then, whether that was really all that Jacob wanted—to go down fighting. I'd be the first to admit that the link to Jacob's fascination with the cinema is circumstantial at best. But when you think about all of the films in which characters make a violent exit in a hail of bullets, perhaps that interpretation isn't so far-fetched.

Some films in this vein, like *Butch Cassidy and the Sundance Kid*, are a simple equation of guns, bullets, and unequal forces that leads to a predictable conclusion. Trapped by hundreds of soldiers, Paul Newman and Robert Redford decide that they'd rather die fighting than be killed, and so they burst out together into a hail of gunfire that ends their lives, and the film. Other films, while not necessarily more believable, carry an equally compelling story. In *Space Cowboys*, for instance, the retired astronaut and barnstorming pilot Hawk Hawkins (Tommy Lee Jones) learns he has inoperable pancreatic cancer and volunteers for what will be a fatal mission. He prefers that end, he says, to a future that would include hospital beds and bedpans.

There's no shortage of other examples that Jacob would have been exposed to, and maybe those films left a mark. Jacob must have recognized that if he wanted to die fighting, the ICU was the only battleground that he had available to him. There weren't going to be any outlaws, gunfights, or final missions. If he wanted a last fight—if that was the way he wanted to be remembered—he was going to have to make do with the plot he had. Not much, perhaps, but enough to make up a credible script in which his cancer was the enemy.

I can't say with certainty whether this was Jacob's real motivation but it is not, in my experience, an uncommon one. I took care of a patient once who had a progressive neurological disease that no one had yet been able to diagnose. A Vietnam veteran, Martin and his wife (and at least one of his doctors) were convinced that his disease was the result of some unidentified chemical exposure during the war. And their conviction motivated what was an interminable and sometimes Kafkaesque battle to force the Veterans Administration to pay for medical care related to his mysterious disease.

When Martin's health began to decline more rapidly near the end of his life, he and his wife faced a sequence of difficult choices about medical treatment. Whether he could remain at home, for instance, or whether he would receive better care in a nursing home. And whether he wanted to go back to the ICU, on one occasion, when he developed a particularly severe form of pneumonia. For each of these choices, and many more, Martin and his wife would talk about his goals and treatment preferences in terms of his identity as a fighter. As in "I've always been a fighter." These weren't boasts and in fact were often deprecatory and self-effacing. "I'm not the sharpest tool in the shed," he'd say, "but I can sure put up a fight."

And these simple statements would lead to anecdotes and, more often, to extended stories that the two of them would adduce as evidence of Martin's identity as a fighter. Only rarely were these stories from the war, though. In fact, I can remember only one, a rather tame administrative scuffle having to do with his promotion that, Martin recalled, was unfairly delayed. Instead, most focused on his illness and on his campaign to receive VA benefits. About how he visited his congressman's office once, sitting in a waiting room for five hours, waiting to plead his case. Or about how he kept working, and even carrying a stool with him to his assembly-line position so that he could continue to work long after most people would have quit.

These examples became signposts, arrayed in a procession along the trajectory of his illness, guiding decisions about his treatment. These examples told Martin and his wife, for instance, that pursuing the most aggressive possible treatment in the ICU was the best choice for someone, like him, who was a fighter. Together, these examples were a heuristic—a rule of thumb—that offered ready guidance for a wide range of medical treatment decisions. In addition, though, these examples were also a constant reminder that Martin and his wife were making the right choices, as long as they were the choices that a fighter would make.

In the end, the signposts that they had been planting so carefully would cease to be useful as guides and would become, instead, constraints that demanded an uncomfortably narrow path for consistency's sake. Eventually, Martin began to experience increasing difficulty breathing on his own and was admitted to the hospital for what was to be the last time. We all knew that there was nothing we could do to slow the progression of his disease, whatever it was, and that a ventilator would only delay his death for a few weeks or a month. Martin and his wife realized this too, as did their daughter, who had come to live with them and had assumed much of the burden of caregiving.

Yet such was the power of those signposts that they'd planted so methodically over the last few years that we all felt compelled to follow the directions that they prescribed. Those signs defined the route that a fighter had taken, and they dictated the course that he should take in the future. And so despite our efforts to reconsider and map out a new route for him, during that final hospitalization Martin, like Jacob, was admitted to the ICU and placed on a ventilator. It wasn't until more than a week later—still in the ICU—that Martin his wife and daughter finally agreed to withdraw treatment.

Martin's story, and his identity as a fighter, is not unusual. In fact, many of my patients take that spirit with them into the fight that they wage with whatever illness has attacked them. But most, I think, eventually concede, as Martin did. They may continue to fight well beyond the point that a victory was possible, but eventually, and often with help from health care providers or family, they're able to reconsider the road map that they've created and to construct a new route that allows a change of direction while preserving their identity. For Martin, what prompted that reconsideration was his family's recognition that the forces arrayed against him were too numerous and too strong, and that, therefore, admitting defeat would not be dishonorable.

Although I don't know whether Jacob thought of himself as a fighter, I do know that others thought of him as one. In fact, I later heard him described by family members and by doctors and nurses who had taken care of him over the years, as "tough" and as "strong-willed," and as a "fighter." None of us in the ICU that night—Steve, Alicia, or I—recognized this motivation explicitly. But I think it had been there, strong enough to help him through the last five years of treatment, and strong enough, ultimately, to shape the final choices that he made that night.

Jacob

If his story had really been written for a film, that night would have been a turning point in Jacob's illness. He would have recovered, left the hospital, gotten married, and perhaps even found a cure after a second bone marrow transplant. But none of us, not even Jacob, imagined that ending. Still, I hoped that we might be able to ensure that Jacob's death would be comfortable, and that he'd be able to spend meaningful time with Marylee and his family.

And for the first few hours after Jacob arrived in the ICU, it looked as though this might be possible. At least we could try to avoid using a ventilator, which would require sedation. But his extended family arrived, and soon it seemed that there was always someone at his bedside, speaking in urgent whispers and probing for a response that would be carried out triumphantly to the waiting room. ("He smiled at the nurse"; "He tried to laugh"; "He said he was doing okay"). Even though these "conversations" were notably one-sided, they soon sapped his energy and he grew increasingly tired. The carbon dioxide levels in his blood began to rise, becoming dangerously high and indicating that he could no longer maintain the effort of breathing on his own. And so just before dawn, as the nursing shift was beginning to change and the rest of the unit was still quiet, we had to do what we had been avoiding all night. We sedated Jacob, inserted an endotracheal tube, and connected the tube to a ventilator.

Jacob's blood gas results improved for a few hours, as we had hoped, but then began to worsen, as we had feared, despite all our efforts to adjust his ventilator settings. A little before noon, his EKG began to show disturbances of his heart rhythm that became increasingly frequent, ending, finally, in a cardiac arrest. Two of the ICU nurses ushered Marylee out into the waiting room as we tried, without any expectations of success, to restart his heart. And that was how Jacob died, receiving all the treatment that we could offer, just as he wanted.

Was this really the death that Jacob wanted? I've often told people his story—or one like it—in hopes that they could help me understand what was motivating Jacob's requests for treatment. Some believe that this ending was exactly what he wanted. Some say this in tones that are admiring or indifferent, but most, I think, are simply stating a fact. There's no accounting for preferences, they seem to suggest, and if that's what Jacob wanted, then that's the way his death needed to be. In fact, this was my initial response as well the day that Jacob died. We did what he asked us to do, I told myself, only partly aware that with this answer I was not defending Jacob's choice so much as I was defending our own response to it.

But others are surprised and confused and see Jacob's death as a mistake. "What did you do wrong?" they ask me. "What else could you have done?" They intuitively sense that this is a horrible death—one that they would have avoided for themselves or their family—and they try to understand how it might have been prevented.

Later, as I put Jacob's death further behind me, I found I was increasingly willing to ask these sorts of questions. And I began to suspect that we could have tried to explore the reasons behind Jacob's requests for treatment. Perhaps we could even have helped him to construct—quickly—a more peaceful alternative to the ending that he had imagined.

Eventually, though, I've come to believe that there are usually no simple answers. And that in Jacob's case there was no single missed opportunity. It's not that we can't learn from stories like Jacob's. And we can certainly try to make sense of the motivations that drive people to pursue every chance of survival. But these motivations are, ultimately, no more than an introduction to thinking about how we die. The real lessons come from those people who consciously turn away from choices that might prolong survival and focus instead on other goals.

TWO

Danny

Parties and Celebrations

Danny

In any medical center there are a few patients—medical celebrities—whose stories seem to gather weight and density spontaneously. They begin as secrets we tell ourselves late at night in deserted hospital cafeterias and cold fluorescent-lit on-call rooms— some, eventually, become legends. And just like legends about celebrities, the patients' tales that become "bestsellers" are those that are able to capture the imagination. Danny's was certainly one of these.

There was a story passed around among the medical residents for six months or so that focused on a man—Danny—who had been diagnosed with advanced cancer. And that diagnosis, we heard, prompted him to trade in a staid and respectable existence for a few final months of reckless abandon. But here the stories diverged widely. According to one account, he had taken up a wildly degenerate life of drinking. According to another, he became a phenomenally successful poker player. Or he bought a motorcycle. Or he lost all of his family's savings at the blackjack table. As most myths are, the permutations of his story were constrained only by the limits of our collective imagination.

Why were these stories so appealing to us? He was portrayed as being young enough that we could all see ourselves in his place in a few more years, so there was that. But there was also the sheer recklessness of his course that, I think, also offered a frisson of living-in-the-moment excitement to overworked and sleep-deprived residents whose lives were carefully arranged exhibits of delayed gratification. Whatever the reason, Danny's story was appealing, attractive, and perfect for an audience like us.

We all recognized, I think, that Danny's story had spread largely through the force of our wanting it to be true. And we knew, therefore, it probably wasn't. So I was surprised when one of my patients told me about a man who seemed to fit the image of Danny that I had imagined.

My patient had had a stroke about a year before and had done exceptionally well. He could speak almost normally and could walk with a cane. But he still had dysphagia—trouble swallowing—and he would choke and cough whenever he tried to drink liquids. So we were talking about a gastrostomy tube, which is a small tube that is introduced directly through the skin into the stomach. I found, though, that I didn't need to provide much detail about the mechanics of how a gastrostomy tube is used. My patient understood immediately.

"It's just like Danny's," he said. "I could win my money back." I didn't recognize "Danny's" name then, and certainly didn't connect my patient's anecdote with the myths I'd heard. Nevertheless, I was intrigued by any tale that could link a gastrostomy tube with gambling. I'd been impressed before this by numerous feats of creative amusement to which Iowans are driven by their long, dark, and bitterly cold winters, and I assumed that I was about to hear about a new one.

Apparently, Danny also had a gastrostomy tube. My patient didn't know why, only that he was "not well," which, in the subdued parlance of Iowa natives, could mean anything from a cold to cancer. Danny had won $20 from my patient (and many other bar patrons, my patient was quick to add) by betting that he could drink a six-pack of beer in a minute. In perpetrating this con, he was abetted by the bartender, who would open a six-pack earlier in the evening, giving it a chance to go flat. Then Danny would solicit bets, identify a few takers, and with a disinterested bystander as a timekeeper, produce a funnel and his gastrostomy tube and pour the contents of the six-pack from a pitcher into his stomach. Even though it left him $20 poorer, my patient thought this trick was really quite spectacular.

I was suspicious at first. Aside from skepticism about feasibility, and ethical concerns about the conditions of the deal—he didn't really "drink" the beer, after all—I found it hard to believe that someone would put a medical device to such a use. So the next time I was in the bar that my patient had mentioned, I asked a bartender about the story. Yes, he had heard it, and yes, it was probably true. But he wasn't party to the deal. That bartender no longer worked there. Besides, the patron hadn't played that trick in a while, although he still stopped by. Perhaps he had used up his potential audience.

The bartender, unfortunately, didn't know much more. But he could give me at least part of Danny's story because he and Danny had both grown up in a small town, West Branch, about ten miles east of Iowa City. A small town in a field of small towns, West Branch was most famous, while I was there at least, for the LB Steakhouse. LB's allowed patrons to grill and butter—with a paintbrush—their own steaks. It was a gimmick that was widely popular and that no doubt contributed modestly to the rates of coronary artery disease and obesity in the county.

The bartender said that Danny had never really been an upstanding citizen. Never an outright criminal, mind you. For instance, he had never done time in jail. The bartender paused for a moment. Well, at least as far as he knew.

But Danny had calmed down over time. He had gotten married, had two kids, and, the bartender thought, his wife had been successful in keeping him in line.

Danny was a part-owner of several small businesses in the city—a pizza place and two newsstands—and owned a couple of tenements that he rented out to students. I must have looked puzzled at this point in the bartender's story. This didn't seem to me to be the type of person who would be making fraternity house–like bets involving large amounts of beer.

Danny, he said, had stayed on something resembling a straight and narrow path until he was in his early forties—about the bartender's age—when he was diagnosed with some kind of abdominal cancer. The bartender wasn't sure. Stomach, maybe. Or liver. But it was bad, that was for sure. Danny went around for a time telling anyone who would listen that he had a year to live. That was about, oh, four or five months ago.

Initially, Danny had been depressed. But depressed in "fits," like he didn't know whether he should be depressed or not. He was a regular at the bar then, and some days he would sit in a corner by himself, drinking deliberately until closing time. Other nights, though, he would make a grand entrance, buy a few rounds for everyone at the bar, leave a big tip for the bartender, and rush off as if he had somewhere to be. Wherever that was, it wasn't his home. Those were the nights Danny's wife would call the bar, asking if Danny was there.

Since then, though, the bartender hadn't seen Danny much. He still came in occasionally, and still bought drinks freely. "But not so crazy now."

Perhaps this tale didn't correspond to the mythical figure we residents had invented. Perhaps that figure had no real-life counterpart at all. Still, the bartender's story was close enough to the legend that I'd heard to let me congratulate myself for a job of sleuthing well done. I was curious to learn more, but not curious enough to try to find Danny, and certainly not curious enough to wait at the bar in ambush. As it turns out, though, I didn't need to. Danny came to me.

Several months later I had forgotten about Danny and my conversation with the bartender when a man in his forties with a history of pancreatic cancer was admitted to me on the gastrointestinal service. He had what appeared to be a near-total obstruction of his common bile duct, which caused profound jaundice but no other symptoms. The diagnosis was easy, as was the treatment—a procedure to place a stent in the bile duct to keep it open. And the intern had already seen him. So I saw half a dozen other new patients first, leaving Danny until last, very late that night.

Because of the way our service was organized, we took care of patients scattered on beds around the hospital, not just on the seventh floor, where the gastrointestinal unit was located. Danny had been given a room four floors down, in the next building over. And so around 3 A.M. I set off, thinking I could talk to Danny and still get an hour or two of sleep before the first calls of the morning began to arrive.

Many of the residents I worked with found the long empty corridors spooky and disconcerting in the middle of the night. But to me they were both comfortable and comforting—as if the enormous hospital had heaved a sigh of relief, expelling almost all of the staff and especially the clipboard-wielding poking and prodding physicians. As I made my way to Danny's unit that night, I was thinking about the magic of the hospital at night, and the benefits, maybe, of taking doctors out of the equation for periods of time.

I wasn't thinking at all about my new patient. His medical care was straightforward and there would be nothing, really, for me to do. If I thought about our impending conversation at all as I walked through the empty halls, it was to wonder with a mild concern how he was going to respond to being woken up by yet another doctor.

But I needn't have worried. I found myself standing in his doorway looking at Danny, who was looking up at me, holding what looked suspiciously like a tumbler of Scotch on the rocks. At least I wouldn't need to wake him up.

Nonplussed, for a moment, I asked him where he got the ice. Even as I spoke, I recognized that my question didn't quite hit the mark. But it was all I could think of.

"A sympathetic nurse." He said this as though it were both obvious and something to be a little proud of.

It was somewhere in that first exchange that the pieces of my patient's history came together for me, although considerably later than they should have. According to his chart, I remembered, he was a small business owner in Iowa City. He had been born and raised nearby and had a wife and two children. He'd been diagnosed with pancreatic cancer about eight months ago. Other pieces of his social history floated back to me and dropped into place, like a history of alcohol abuse and the impressions of several previous physicians that he was manipulative. It all fit.

I stood in the doorway, finally staring at the man who, I guessed, I had heard so much about. Strangely, he was more or less what I expected. Sitting on the edge of the hospital bed, resting his elbows on the rolling table in front of him, he could have been back at his favorite bar. He was short and stocky, with beefy arms connected seamlessly to sloping shoulders, a thick bull neck, and a shovel jaw. He looked, I thought, like some yet-to-be-invented piece of heavy construction machinery. The kind you'd use to tear up tree stumps, maybe, or to level a wall.

"The bar's open. Want a drink? Johnny Walker Black—the best."

He seemed so much at home, and his invitation seemed so natural, that I almost forgot for a moment that I was a doctor and he was a patient. A patient—my patient—who shouldn't be drinking anything a few hours before a surgical procedure. But I didn't want to argue with him. There would be time enough for that later. Instead, I was curious to find out whether, in fact, this was the man I had heard so much about.

So I didn't accept or refuse. Instead, I edged into the room and sat down on the empty bed across from him. I asked him how he was doing.

"What do you mean?"

Now I was on more solid ground. I had been thinking about Danny's case so much, albeit in the back of my mind, that my questions seemed to form themselves.

"I mean that you've been through a lot in the last year. A bad diagnosis. G-tube. And at least one other bile duct obstruction like the one that brought you here tonight. You've been in the hospital how many times in the last few months? Five? Ten?"

"I'm not counting. Time in the hospital doesn't matter. It's just time away from real life."

His answer sounded dismissive, yet something I'd said had gotten his attention. He was looking at me with a new appreciation, and just a touch of curiosity, as if he wanted to see where this conversation was going to lead.

"OK, so tell me about your real life. How is that going?"

"Why do you want to know about my real life? You're a doctor, this is your world." He waved a thick hand at the institutional hospital furniture, the row of valves for oxygen and suction on the walls, and the empty bed I was sitting on.

"You, and them"—he gestured at the nursing station—"you just worry about what goes on in here. My life is my business."

There were a number of possible responses to this. Foremost of which was the observation that it was largely his life "out there," like his drinking, which was responsible for at least some of his time "in here." But I didn't think an argument about his lifestyle would get us anywhere. So I just said what I was thinking.

"I'm just curious. I'm wondering how everything you've been through has changed your life out there. It must have, right?" I was fishing a bit. But also genuinely curious.

He was quiet for a moment. Ruminative, but watchful. As I waited for an answer to form, I noticed that he didn't really have the hard, bulldozing appearance that I thought I'd seen from the door. He seemed diminished now. His arms were heavy, but his shoulders were smaller than they used to be, to judge from the extra folds of his Hawaiian print shirt. And what had seemed like a barrel chest tenting his shirtfront was actually a belly swollen from ascites—fluid that had built up because of the obstruction caused by his cancer. But what struck me most after those first few minutes was that his confidence, including his initial offer of a drink to me, was thin and fragile. I suspected then that if I were to grab his tumbler and toss his Scotch in the sink behind me, he might not protest too much.

So he told me about his "real" life and about how he'd been spending the last few months. As he did, it seemed to me that he was mostly bragging. For instance, he told me about the drinking I already knew about, as well as a lot of gambling I didn't. "I blew a thousand bucks at the riverboats on craps in one night. Since I was so far behind, I gave the croupier a hundred, and a fifty each to the table girls. They'll sure remember me next time."

That was true. And perhaps they would even remember him as generous. Or perhaps, I thought, they would laugh at a hapless loser who couldn't lose his money fast enough and so began to give it away. I said his life didn't really sound so good to me.

But it was, he said. He was having a grand time. This was really living.

It was already very late, and I had spent too much time with what should have been a routine admission. More than half an hour, so far, when a nod from the doorway would have been sufficient. With a bit of luck, I could still get a few hours of sleep before the morning lab results started to come in, prompting urgent calls from the nurses' station. On the other hand, I was no closer, really, to understanding why Danny was throwing away his time and his family's money at bars and casinos.

And it had also become obvious to me that at least some of Danny's behavior was self-destructive. This wasn't just a harmless fling, sprinkled with small-time gambling and bar tricks. His drinking was certainly affecting his health, and his gambling must have been a financial burden to his family. So I resolved to try, at least, to figure out what was driving Danny.

Explaining the Pursuit of Pleasure at the End of Life

If I suspected that night that Danny's behavior was both self-destructive and wrong, I also had a vague sense that it wasn't entirely unusual. Even then, as I sat listening to Danny the raconteur, I could think of a few historical examples that were, if anything, more extreme. For instance, I dimly remembered an account I had read years before of the cholera epidemic that settled over Naples in 1884. A few days after I met Danny, I was able to find the passage I had remembered from a somewhat fictionalized autobiography of the Swedish physician Axel Munthe.

> *Sodom and Gomorrah were nothing compared to Naples. Did I not see what was going on in the poor quarters, in the streets, in the infected houses, even in the churches while they were praying to one saint and cursing another? A frenzy of lust was sweeping all over Naples, immorality and vice everywhere in the very face of Death.*

Munthe's description is a bit overwrought. It seems unlikely to me that an epidemic disease whose primary symptom is copious diarrhea could produce the city-wide bacchanal that Munthe describes. A frenzy of lust, indeed.

Yet his account is not wholly unbelievable, and in fact I thought of another example as Danny and I sat there. It was a painting I had seen in the Louvre years before of a shipwreck off the coast of—I thought—South America that ended in a wild frenzy of drinking and violence. When I was able to find that story much later, my memory of the wreck itself proved to be faulty. Nevertheless, the chaos that ensued proved to be even more dramatic than I had remembered it.

When the *Méduse* sank in 1816 off the coast of Africa (not South America) over 150 people were left on a raft stitched together from the ship's spars, supplied with only three casks of wine and two of water. On their second night afloat, a group of sailors and soldiers became convinced that the end was near and commandeered one of the wine casks. That wine, shared out among perhaps a dozen men, was enough to start a drunken brawl that lasted the rest of the night and destroyed all of their remaining water and wine. The grotesque painting of the aftermath of this rampage that I remembered from the Louvre, known in English as *The Raft of the Medusa*, was by Théodore Géricault and was informed, it turns out, by Géricault's interviews with two of the survivors.

These examples, or at least my imperfect recollections of them, both distorted and gave life to the way that I listened to the story that Danny told me that night. On one hand, the admittedly superficial similarities between Danny's own behavior and Munthe's and Géricault's descriptions of lust and drunkenness were hardly flattering. And so these examples reinforced the reservations I had had about the way Danny was acting.

On the other hand—and this is more difficult to explain—the fact that these examples involved dozens if not hundreds of people suggested that, in choosing to drink and gamble through his final months, at least Danny had company. Not good company, certainly, but company nonetheless. And so I was perhaps not as quick as I might have been to dismiss his behavior as boorish and crude, viewing it instead with a vague distaste tinged with a sort of prurient curiosity.

I wondered, in fact, how many of us would behave like Danny if we found ourselves in his circumstances. Or like the drunken group of soldiers and sailors from the *Méduse,* or like the people in Munthe's description of the inhabitants of Naples. Why not spend your time embracing at least a few of the more harmless cardinal sins? If you set aside for a moment the impact that Danny's behavior had on his family and look at what he was doing in isolation, was it really that awful?

I wasn't prepared to answer any of these questions that night. But, thinking of those historical accounts, I was more willing than I might otherwise have been to think of Danny not as an anomaly—a deviant—but as someone who was following a path that many others had pursued before him. And it was that realization, more than anything, that kept me in the room with Danny, trying to figure out what, exactly, was driving him.

Distraction

My first thought, as Danny and I surveyed one another, was that he was looking for an escape. He was looking for something—any-thing—that would distract his attention from his illness and prog-nosis. This seemed so obvious an explanation, in fact, that I had difficulty imagining any other. Given Danny's diagnosis, who among us wouldn't want to find some respite?

Faced with a terminal illness, it seems natural to want to escape the burden of knowing that we have only a few months more to live. And to avoid, for a while at least, our fears of the pain and suffering that those last few months might bring. In fact, for almost all of my patients I'm convinced that some escape through distraction is at least appealing and perhaps even necessary.

Nor is that desire for escape limited to patients facing a terminal illness. I'm thinking, for instance, of the letters between death-row inmates and those who write to them. According to many of these volunteers that I've met, a consistent theme seems to be the way their letters remind inmates of what it's like to lead a normal life. Jo Williamson, who also happens to be a hospice worker, told me that her pen friends often find relief in her stories of everyday life. "Any-thing," she said, "that will distract them from their circumstances for a short while."

And this theme, or something like it, appears in many of the letters from death row that Jan Arriens has collected over years of correspondence. These are letters from inmates like Andrew Lee Jones, who wrote shortly before he was executed in Louisiana in July of 1991: "Since I have been writing to you the thought of dying in the electric chair don't cross my mind too much because I have a lot to think about when you write. With your letters and pictures I can put myself on a hill, I can run wild on a Scottish island. I can take my mind completely out of this place."

So it seems to me that a desire for escape exists in a wide range of circumstances, from a death sentence to a terminal diagnosis. Yet when my patients seek out activities that could provide distraction, I almost always face hesitant and uncertain questions from their family members or health care providers. However natural a desire for escape may be, there is apparently something deeply disconcerting about the disengagement that results.

I once took care of a teenager who had recently received a diagnosis of a craniopharyngioma, a particularly aggressive, and deadly, form of cancer that involves the sinuses and upper airway. Clara had been through an intensive program of surgery, radiation, and chemotherapy, but her tumor had recurred, even further advanced now than it had been when first discovered. Throughout that hospitalization, all day, every day, her room remained dark, with the curtains closed. Day and night, her television stayed on, a constant presence that she would watch steadily, engulfed by its bluish light that spread through her room and spilled out into the hall.

When I went in to talk with her in the morning, at seven o'clock or even earlier, the television was already on, or still on, with the sound turned down. Sometimes, Clara was dozing, but usually she was awake, stony-faced, hypnotized by whatever scene was playing out at the foot of her bed. It seemed that she had access to an endless supply of movies—from friends, family, and a devoted hospital volunteer—that were stacked on her bedside table like an improvised wall. She would watch movies all night, the nurses told me, dozing intermittently. But even when she fell asleep, they said, she would never rewind the film to see whatever she had missed. It was as if she needed a trancelike immersion in those images as they spooled by, without knowing or caring what had come before.

Those of us who were taking care of Clara were in turns frustrated, confused, and finally concerned. It was as if she'd chosen to remain sedated, deep in an anesthesia of fantasy, for whatever time she had left. Whenever I came into her room, for instance, it was difficult if not impossible to get her attention. She was never rude, and she'd respond to direct questions. But even when she turned to look at me, it was obvious that her attention was being pulled away by the images flickering at the edge of her field of vision.

Her mother, too, was worriedly apologetic. This wasn't like Clara, she said. What was wrong with her? She needed to wake up and fight this cancer. So her mother had her own vision of what Clara should be doing—fighting—that was driven by her own fears of losing her daughter.

But her mother's urgings had an odd, galvanizing effect on all of us. Even though she was echoing our own concerns, there was something about her directness that made us more sympathetic to Clara's needs. And so we found ourselves siding with Clara. She's been through a lot, we said. She needs time. She needs to rest and collect her strength. We made excuses for her even as we worried quietly among ourselves, because we needed Clara to be an active participant—a partner—in decisions about her treatment.

But I wasn't sure what role Clara wanted, or needed, to play. It was almost as if she was letting others—Clint Eastwood, Sylvester Stallone, Mel Gibson—fight a battle on her behalf. They would win, or perhaps they would lose. And she would remain safe in the stands as an onlooker.

After Clara went home with hospice care, we learned that she did begin to open up, spending more time with her family and even taking a role in planning her memorial service with her best friend and her two sisters. But throughout the next seven weeks until her death, whenever the world overwhelmed her, Clara would retreat to her room, where her hospice nurse would find her, as I had seen her last, keeping a quiet sort of company with Sylvester Stallone.

The medical profession has only begun to realize what Clara seemed to understand intuitively, that there is a therapeutic value to the rest and respite that distraction offers. In hospice in particular, there has been a growing recognition that many forms of complementary medicine offer distraction and relief. Music therapy, art therapy, and even massage therapy all offer an escape for a few minutes from difficult circumstances. Family members, too, and even hospice staff, find value in these sorts of therapies.

But sources of distraction need not be complicated. Indeed, I've often wondered whether many of the activities that take up my patients' time offer a similar mechanism of distraction. Sorting papers, for instance, and organizing possessions. When my grandmother became more frail, for instance, she began to sort through old photo albums and boxes of carefully packed china and glassware, making sure that every item that deserved a home found one within the family. Of course, this sorting wasn't only a source of distraction. But there was, I think, a reassuring solidity in the process. It was neither physically nor cognitively demanding, but it was engaging. Engaging enough, I think, to provide form and structure to her time, and just demanding enough to help her forget her own failing health.

On the other hand, though, sometimes what appears to be a desire for distraction is much simpler, and almost reflexive. Sister Helen Prejean tells a wonderful story about one of her last conversations with Patrick Sonnier before he was executed. She was surprised, she says, and even uncomfortable, as the two of them sat quietly talking of rabbit hunting, tracking, and ways of preparing venison when Sonnier was only a day away from death. In that simple anecdote, theories about denial, distraction, and other motivations seem abstract—not so much wrong as beside the point.

Sonnier didn't talk about hunting because he wanted to avoid talking about his execution, Sister Helen decided. It just wasn't possible for him, and perhaps for anyone, to focus exclusively on death and dying. "You can only attend to death for so long," she wrote, "before the life force sucks you right in again." I don't think she is being particularly mystical here. When pleasurable thoughts are so tightly connected to family, home, and other aspects of life that are meaningful, they're impossible to set aside, no matter how dire the circumstances.

You can see this, or something like it, in the waiting rooms of intensive care units and in hospice family lounges. Or walk down the halls of any hospice unit and peek into the patient rooms. A few rooms will be stifled by the thick, twilit silence of the deathbed scene you'd expect. From others, though, and perhaps the majority, you'll hear the rumble of adult conversations, the rattle of children's voices, and even laughter.

But Danny's behavior seemed to be on another level entirely. His drinking and gambling couldn't really be explained simply by irrepressible energy. No, he must have been hoping that the fleeting camaraderie of the bar and the excitement of the craps table would take his mind off his condition and his future, I thought. And the steady drip of alcohol, too, must surely have helped. Together, maybe those pursuits gave him the same sort of respite that Clara found in her movies.

Remembrance of Things Past

Of course, there was a difference between Danny's behavior and Clara's. For Clara, that television screen in a darkened room offered a pure form of escape. It didn't seem to matter which film was playing. As long as its plot had sufficient action to capture and hold her attention, any film would do.

But Danny didn't seem to be looking only for an escape from the confines of a terminal illness or a respite from the pressure of a dismal prognosis. Instead, he seemed to be driven by some sort of vision. In his raucous life "out there" he seemed to be looking for something. But what?

I took care of a patient once who began to drink and gamble near the end of his life in a way that reminded me more than a little of Danny. Richard had extremely fragile health due to a variety of diagnoses, including heart failure, emphysema, and peripheral vascular disease. He wouldn't have met most people's definitions of "terminally ill." But I knew that he would become increasingly weak and frail until, at some point, he would suffer some catastrophic event—a heart attack, stroke, pneumonia—that would kill him.

Over the six months or so that I knew him, Richard gradually lost the ability to walk independently. That loss left him unable to do his own shopping and made him frustratingly dependent on his son and his daughter-in-law. And his frailty and decline were especially difficult for Richard because he had always lived, more than most of us do, in the physical world.

He had worked in construction all his life and, he told me proudly, he'd even helped to build the hospital where I worked. After he retired, he maintained the same active life, but now doing the things that he'd always wanted to do. He bought a part-ownership in a deep-sea charter boat, for instance, and went out for days at a time helping clients to land bluefish in the summer, yellowfin and bluefin in the fall, and sea bass throughout the winter. And he bought several houses in his neighborhood and renovated them with his son. This active, physical life was, for him, the good life.

And so, more than it would have been for most of us, the loss of that physical life was devastating. As he lost the ability to handle the fishing boat and to climb a ladder, he began, inexplicably, to spend long weekends drinking and gambling in Atlantic City. Sometimes he would go with friends, but often he would go alone.

I only learned about these trips from Richard's son, who had become concerned that his father was drinking too much. I was reluctant to intervene, though. From what I could tell, these weekends didn't seem to be affecting Richard's health, and the amounts of money that he seemed to be spending were modest. Without realizing it, I suppose that Danny had become my yardstick against which pleasure and debauchery were measured. By that standard, at least, Richard's behavior was so tame as to be almost unnoticeable.

But Richard's son was persistent, and so finally I asked Richard why he went on his trips. He gave me an honest answer, although I didn't recognize it at first. He said, in essence, that sitting at the craps table gave him energy.

At first I thought he meant that literally. I thought he meant that Atlantic City was a stimulating environment that let him overcome, if only for a night, the fatigue and frailty that had come to constrict his life. And my impression was strengthened by the way that Richard became animated as he tried to explain his trips. He seemed twenty years younger—vital, confident, and hopeful.

I still didn't understand Richard's trips any more than his son did, but Richard obviously loved to talk about them. So I'd ask him about his latest adventure whenever he came to the clinic. And those stories—brief anecdotes, really—gave a much more accurate picture of what really motivated him.

I realized eventually that Richard wasn't drawn to the casinos just to dip into the energy and excitement that they generated. More important to him, I think, was the way those feelings brought back memories of past raucous weekends there. I began to appreciate these memories as, in Richard's telling, a brief story of the past weekend would reliably segue into a longer—and probably embellished—story of a weekend years ago. Like the time he and his buddies spent five nights in Atlantic City after they had just finished a particularly long job and were flush with cash.

Perhaps those memories were enhanced by the excitement of gambling and by the pleasant sensation of a few complimentary drinks. Still, those trips to Atlantic City weren't so much about the pleasure of drinking and gambling, nor were they simply a distraction. More than anything, they were a memory aid of sorts, helping him to recall and relive his past. Those weekends were to Richard, I suppose, more or less what madeleines were to Proust.

And so I wonder whether something like this was driving Danny as well. Perhaps the time he spent in bars and at the casinos put him in touch, at least temporarily, with memories of an earlier period of his life, one in which he was healthy and hopeful. He was no longer that person any more than Richard was. Like Richard, he knew that the person he had been—aggressive, independent, healthy—was gone. But for both men, maybe, their nights in the bars and casinos gave them a chance to reexperience what it felt like to be that person.

Celebration

Sometimes pleasure is neither a distraction nor a way of recapturing a past experience but is simply the foundation—or the excuse—for a celebration. It was a friend and colleague, Ira Byock, who pointed this out to me. Sometimes, he said, what seems like a pursuit of pleasure, or distraction, is really a celebration of someone's life, their accomplishments, and their relationships.

One of the best-known final celebrations occurs in the account of Socrates' final hours in the *Phaedo*. Socrates, Plato tells us, gathered his friends and disciples for one final celebration before he drank his prescribed hemlock. It's noteworthy, perhaps, that Socrates, like Danny, appears to have sent his wife and family away, preferring to spend his time with his friends. And while that choice is less than admirable, I've always loved Socrates' example, even more so because it comes from a hardheaded proponent of reason and logic. That this celebration seems out of character, at least to me, makes it all the more appealing.

For Carlos, though, an older Puerto Rican man with advanced heart failure who stealthily orchestrated what was to be his last party, a final celebration was utterly in character. Over the past few months he had been in and out of the hospital several times for exacerbations of his heart failure, each episode leaving him progressively weaker and more frail. At least one of those hospitalizations, I knew, had been precipitated by a heart attack that Carlos had either not been aware of or, more likely, had simply ignored.

Shortly after Carlos was admitted the final time, his cardiologist had done an angiogram—a dye study of his heart—to try to find one or two coronary arteries that might be opened with a balloon catheter. But she found, instead, significant narrowing of all the large arteries that feed the heart, narrowing that was too diffuse, and too advanced, to try to open or to bypass using surgery. The best we could do, she told me, would be to find a combination of medications that would keep Carlos out of trouble for a little while longer.

That news came at a particularly unfortunate time. Carlos's hospitalization coincided with a massive visit of a sister and three brothers and most of their children, which had been planned almost a year in advance to celebrate the thirtieth anniversary of his move to Iowa (a few months early) and his seventieth birthday (a few weeks late). His family had reserved a pavilion at a state park nearby, and had levied accommodations from friends and neighbors (all of whom were also invited). And they'd begun cooking, it seemed, weeks in advance.

I learned all this from one of Carlos's nieces who lived in Iowa City, where she was enrolled in medical school. I walked in on a heated discussion in rapid-fire Spanish between her and Carlos in which, as near as I could tell, Carlos was insisting that the party should proceed as planned. But his niece was trying to explain—timidly yet firmly—that she had already started to postpone it.

She appealed to me. Wasn't Carlos too sick for a party? his niece asked. "*¿Esta muy grave, no?*"—"He's seriously ill, isn't he?" Carlos's niece spoke English fluently, but the Spanish was for Carlos's benefit, to be sure that no word would be lost. A celebration might kill him, she insisted. Carlos simply shrugged. They had, I guessed, been over this ground many times before.

Carlos switched to a fluent English for me, perhaps hoping that I would take his side. I deserved this party a week ago, he said slyly. Now I don't deserve it anymore? What did I do to make my family so angry with me that they won't even come to my party?

His niece threw her hands skyward, exasperated, in a gesture that didn't require a translation. They both turned to look at me, and I thought for a panicked moment that they wanted me to adjudicate. But then they turned back to each other and switched to a rapid Spanish that I could barely follow.

They weren't in need of a mediator, I thought, just an audience. So I concentrated on Carlos's physical examination, made considerably more difficult and even somewhat hazardous by his frequent gesticulations. I finished the exam, noting that his weight had increased since the previous day, a sign that he was becoming fluid-overloaded again. Eventually, I retreated, my departure barely noticed by either Carlos or his niece.

I was on call that day and my responsibilities took me elsewhere in the hospital for a while. But in my absence, somehow, a Saturday afternoon visit by a few family members turned into a gathering of the entire extended family. Soon nephews and cousins spilled out into the hallway and, eventually, into the family meeting room at the end of the hall.

From somewhere, a casserole dish of pork and rice and beans a caballo (with a layer of fried eggs on top) appeared, accompanied by forks and paper plates and napkins scavenged from the cafeteria downstairs. And then, through some biblical catering mechanism, that single casserole was transformed into a heavily laden table—of almojabanas (fritters stuffed with chicken), baked batatas (sweet potatoes), and mondongo, a beef stew whose ingredients one of the cousins described vividly—if unhelpfully—as "cow pieces." When a radio appeared, there were mutterings at the nurses' station, but those were quickly quieted when a tray of besito de coco, a dessert of shaved coconut and sugar, appeared in the nurses' break room.

The celebration was just gathering momentum early that afternoon, when a new admission brought me back to Carlos's ward. Increasingly curious, and more than a little hungry, I stopped by perhaps two or three times that day to watch his party unfold. Every time, as I stood in the doorway of the family room, that vibrant mix of laughing and talking, mingled with the smell of cilantro and onions and garlic and the sounds of festive *danzas* would wash out into the hall.

But what I remember most of that long summer afternoon were the glimpses I got of Carlos himself. I was surprised to see that he wasn't at the center of the party, and he didn't even seem to be an active participant. He was in a wheelchair up against one wall of the room, leaving the floor clear for the spinning children. Yet every time I saw him, he was watching, nodding, and smiling. A wide, all-encompassing smile that flickered just a bit as he dipped his head subtly in time to the music. He looked peaceful but intensely, completely satisfied, as if all of his life had led inexorably to this one perfect moment.

And in a way, it had. He was surrounded by examples of all that he had accomplished. A cousin who could afford to come to Iowa because his gas station, begun with Carlo's investment, had been so successful. His nephew, who everyone said would be a star soccer player someday because Carlos saw his nascent talent and insisted on paying to send him to an elite soccer camp. And Carlos's niece, now in her second year of medical school because Carlos had pushed her to be the first doctor in the family. Everyone in that room was evidence of the life that he had led. They were proof of what he had created and what he had done. And their presence there, that afternoon, was the best possible celebration of his life.

Did Carlos realize this celebration would be his last? I'm sure he knew he didn't have much time left. His cardiologist and I both had had that conversation with him, and Carlos's niece had certainly done her best to convince him that he was seriously ill. Besides, the experience of the angiogram and the pictures of his heart and his blocked arteries that we showed him would have left little room for irrational optimism. And yet, in vivid contrast to that bleak photograph of his threadlike coronary arteries, Carlos was very much alive that afternoon.

Perhaps he was hopeful that he might live to see a few more parties in the future. When I came back to see him later that evening, after the party had broken up, I was surprised to find him eating dinner. Surely a hospital tray couldn't compare to his cousins' cooking? Carlos sighed. He hadn't eaten anything at the party, he said. Too much adobo, a salt-laced all-purpose seasoning. He had to take care of himself, he said.

Carlos did take care of himself, at least for a time. He returned home, with family and neighbors stopping by to check on him. He lived at home for another month or so until he became weaker and moved in with one of his cousins. He enrolled in hospice not long afterward and died without another trip to the hospital.

I still think of Carlos's as the perfect celebration, in part because his "guests" could join in various ways. For the children—and there seemed to be dozens—it was a party. For most of the others, it was a congratulatory celebration of Carlos's life, and a chance to thank him for all that he had done for the family. And for a few, like his niece, who appreciated the seriousness of the latest hospitalization, this was a celebration of the end of his life. But—and this is the most important part—a somber acknowledgment that Carlos was dying wasn't a precondition of participation. Everyone there was celebrating, with Carlos, in a slightly different way.

And Carlos's party was perfect, too, because it was timed so well. His celebration happened early enough that he was still engaged in life and living. Yet he was seriously ill enough that the nearness of death conferred a sense of importance and singularity to what might otherwise have seemed spontaneous and or even frivolous.

This perfect timing, of course, can be elusive. I heard once about a celebration, organized by the wife of a man who was enrolled in hospice, which was a phenomenal success. It was so well received, in fact, that when the man was still alive several months later, though still seriously ill, the only appropriate response seemed to be another party. He died shortly after the second celebration. I like to think that these events could have gone on for years, and perhaps they might have begun much earlier. A celebration could become as much a part of dying as updating and revising one's will. It would be an event to be arranged regularly, not in anticipation of death but rather as a hedge against it.

These are wonderful examples—Carlos's especially—but I'm afraid their glow doesn't shed much light on Danny's motivations. Danny's pursuit of pleasure seemed to me to be solitary, boorish, and almost misanthropic. There were elements of his story, of course, that had the sheen of camaraderie, like the evenings spent in the loose fellowship of a bar. But I don't really think there was any true friendship there. Nor, really, was there anything like a celebration.

There could have been, though. Danny was nothing if not gregarious, and he could be witty and charming, his nurse told me later, particularly when he wanted something. And so if he had wanted to create a celebration, I'm certain it would have been a grand one.

Final Adventures

Through the twists and turns of my conversation with Danny that night, I'd caught no more than a glimpse of his motivation. I looked surreptitiously at my watch and was surprised to see that we'd been talking for over an hour. Yet I was still no closer to understanding Danny's motivation than I had been when I'd first heard his story from the bartender. And I probably never would have if I hadn't asked him how his wife felt about his behavior. The long nights out, the drinking and gambling. Did she mind?

"She doesn't mind me being crazy for a while," he said with what sounded like a very thin sort of courage. At least, she had told him, until "I get it out of my system."

I must have looked confused because he continued, after a pause, explaining that after his diagnosis he felt that there were things that he had missed. He should be doing more. He was past forty and had lived his entire life in Iowa City, or nearby. The move from West Branch to Iowa City, in fact, had been the big adventure in his life. He didn't think that was much. He felt like he still had more living to do. What he really wanted, he said, was to try on a different, more interesting life for a while. It was now or never.

So what kind of life would he want?

What he really wanted, he said, was a "large" life in a city like Chicago. A Porsche, a girlfriend (or two), a loft on Michigan Avenue, and a speedboat to play with on the weekends. "That's the kind of man I could have been. I could've been able to buy all that."

And that, it turned out, was Danny's simple secret. His father had developed a progressive lung disease when Danny was a senior in high school. So Danny gave up plans to go to college and business school, instead staying at home working to support his parents. He started out at one of the large multipurpose supply stores out on Route 6, run by a friend of his father's, but he never got a promotion, and eventually moved on to other jobs.

He'd been good at selling things, he said. Insurance, cars, and restaurant products, for instance. But he'd never had the tenacity to stick to anything for more than a year. Most sideways ventures didn't pay off, but a few did. And after two decades of minor gains and many setbacks, he came to own parts of a few businesses and some property. He was successful by Iowa City standards, and an over-achiever by the standards of his small hometown. But he fell far short of what he thought he should be.

So Danny had carried a vision of the person he could have been around with him ever since his father died, like you might carry a worn picture of a long-lost brother stashed in a wallet. I don't think Danny was really trying to become that person. It seems more likely that he wanted to feel what it would be like to be that person, for a brief period of time. He wanted to experience the sense of power, or influence, or admiration, that person would have experienced every day. But he was realistic enough to recognize, certainly, that he wasn't that person, and that he never would be.

If that seems a tenuous dichotomy, supported by a fragile suspension of disbelief, I don't think it's at all unusual. In medical school I took care of a girl in her teens with cystic fibrosis, a chronic and incurable inherited lung disease. Back then, treatments were more limited than they are now and lung transplants—the current cure—were still experimental. Moreover, she had a particularly severe form of the disease, which she knew would probably kill her before she turned eighteen. And with that appreciation of her prognosis came the realization that her dream of becoming an airline pilot was finally and irrevocably out of reach.

Still, she wanted to have that experience. She wanted to know what it feels like to sit in a plane's cockpit, helping run through the preflight checklist, talking with her copilot on a headset. And maybe, if she were lucky, to watch the white lines of the runway fly beneath the plane as the plane tipped up and the ground receded. But—and this is the most important point—she knew that she would not actually be flying the plane and that she would never be a pilot.

As far as I know, she never got that wish, despite the best efforts of our social worker. There had been, we heard, an anesthesia resident at our hospital who had a pilot's license, but he had left. There was a flight school that might help, but they would charge a fee that the girl's parents couldn't afford. And, too, there were medical obstacles. It was these concerns about her breathing and need for oxygen that finally ended our attempts to arrange a flight for her.

Other children are more fortunate, particularly those who find their way to an organization like the Make-A-Wish Foundation. Their staff and volunteers have become adept at overcoming the sorts of barriers that blocked our efforts to put my patient in the cockpit of a plane. Volunteers, for instance, who arranged a Sweet Seventeen party for a girl with a congenital heart defect whose illness had made a more traditional Sweet Sixteen party impossible. Or those who, somehow, managed to obtain a small part for another girl in a major studio film *(The Princess Diaries)*. Some wishes are easier to arrange, of course, like those of Markell, a seven-year-old boy with sickle-cell anemia whose wish was to ride a horse, or of John, a fifteen-year-old boy with an autoimmune disease who wanted to take his friends swimming at a local pool.

These stories of children are wonderfully uplifting, but I find the stories of adults to be even more compelling. Whereas children have been denied experiences like flying a plane by their illnesses, my patients—adults—have been denied these experiences at least in part because of choices they made. Danny, for instance, could have gone back to school, and he could have moved to a larger city. But he didn't, and so the last few months of his life offered a chance to try to see what his life might have been like if he had made different choices twenty years earlier. There is a compelling pathos that drives, and funds, organizations whose sole purpose is to grant the wishes of children. But it's too bad that there aren't organizations with equivalent resources for adults—organizations that would rally to provide people like Danny with the experiences that they should have had.

Perhaps it's ludicrous to imagine any sort of organized experience that would have let Danny live, for a while, the dream life that he had imagined. What he wanted was not an experience so much as it was an identity. And perhaps an experience inspired by that life—a weekend in Chicago, or a weeklong executive internship at a brokerage firm—would simply reinforce rather than relieve Danny's regrets about the life that he could have had. He would see it, immediately, as the cheap substitute that it was.

Still, perhaps he could have simply enjoyed the experience, setting aside dreams and regrets. And wasn't this, really, what Danny had been doing in the year before I met him? Surely he had spent enough time imagining that life to know, in minute detail, what it should look like. And just as surely he would have recognized a counterfeit. He must have recognized that the role he was acting out was, at best, a diluted version of who he wanted to be.

So perhaps a fairer interpretation is that Danny recognized that the role he was playing was not, in fact, taken directly from the life that he felt he had been denied. He must have realized this just as clearly as my patient with cystic fibrosis recognized that she would never be an airplane pilot. But this role was close enough to give him a sense—albeit distorted, and above all transient—of what he might have experienced if his life had taken a different course.

Freedom

It was surprising to me, that night, how far off course Danny had veered in the space of a few months. At the time of his diagnosis, Danny was a solid businessman. Not long before he'd been a father, husband, and property owner. But he had jumped the tracks and was racing across country in a wild dash to . . . somewhere.

What was so astonishing to me then, and what still surprises me now, is that no one did anything to stop him. Not his friends, not his wife, and certainly not the croupier and cocktail waitresses at the riverboat casinos who looked forward to spending Danny's children's college fund. Not even me.

But I shouldn't have been surprised. We tend to accord considerable freedom to people near the end of life. Indeed, many of the other examples in this chapter—Clara, Richard, Carlos—are evidence of this. Just as Danny's wife gave him the freedom he thought he needed, we all empathized with Clara's escape in front of her television. And Carlos's niece backed down sooner than she might have otherwise, letting him have the party he wanted. And even though Richard's son was concerned about Richard's trips to the casinos, he never tried to prevent them.

Tying all of these examples together is a sort of unquestioning permissiveness that we grant to those near the end of life. It is, ultimately, a sort of global dispensation. Sometimes the result is a new freedom that is conferred in picturesque ways. In what has become a classic ethnographic study, Myra Bluebond-Langner describes in minute detail the freedoms that children dying of cancer were accorded by parents and health care providers. For instance, one boy received his Christmas presents in October. And another who wanted a winter coat was allowed to buy one in July.

Sometimes these freedoms are granted, and even institution-alized, in bizarre forms. Consider, for instance, the tradition of a "last meal" that is eaten, and supposedly enjoyed, by a condemned prisoner just hours before his or her execution. The rites and lore that have grown around this simple tradition are macabre, sad, and funny at the same time. Accounts from the last hours of death-row inmates include stories of meals that are wildly improbable, both in terms of their choices and, sometimes, their sheer volume. Plat-ters of chicken fried steak, hamburgers, turkey and gravy, and ice-cream sundaes, all served to people who will be dead in a few hours. These accounts read like a culinary black comedy in which the inmates seem to be following a script that is thrust on them by the prison staff, who are compelled to respond to the inmate's wishes.

Viewed against the backdrop of these examples, perhaps the freedom that Danny enjoyed is not so remarkable. Nevertheless, it's too bad that he was accorded this freedom without any constraint or guidance. Perhaps with the right advice he might have made more of the time he had. Or at least he might have used his freedom in a way that was less destructive.

Danny

After almost two hours of rambling conversation, I'd eventually begun to see Danny's wild behavior as a sort of striving after an ex-perience that he felt he had missed. There would be elements that fell into place later, and bits of his story that I would learn from others who had taken care of him. But I felt that I had at least a general explanation. Enough, I thought. Besides, it was almost 5 A.M. I was tempted to beat a retreat and to get an hour or two of sleep.

On the other hand, I didn't feel like I could walk away from such a misguided plan. I wasn't sure that what Danny was doing was wrong, but I was convinced that I should at least raise the possibility that it might be. If the rest of Danny's life were in order, I thought, and he had no family to think about, then I couldn't criticize him for wanting to capture whatever experiences he seemed to think he had missed. But that was hardly the case.

Danny had a wife and children who were probably hurt by his prolonged absence. At the very least his children were missing a valuable opportunity to spend time with him. And then, of course, there was the financial harm that Danny's gambling was inflicting on his family.

So I asked him, tentatively, whether there might be better ways he could use his time. He was silent for a moment. But just a moment. And as he began to answer, I realized that mine was a question that he'd probably heard before and was perhaps even one that he was waiting for. If he expected my question, I certainly hadn't anticipated his response to me.

So I thought he had been an asshole? he asked. Said as a challenge, it sounded to me more like an honest question. A question of fact, even, the sort a patient might ask me about whether a mole might be malignant or an irregular heart rhythm might be cause for concern.

I couldn't believe we were having this discussion, but why not? Well, yes, as a matter of fact, I did think he had been an asshole. And I proceeded to list everything that he had done that I thought qualified. He took money from his family's bank account. He used that money to drink and gamble. He missed the chance to see his daughter in her prom dress because he was at a bar. This last jab was a guess based on what I had heard from the bartender, but it seemed to strike home.

"OK, OK, I've got it. I'm an asshole." He paused. "But I really want to lead the good life while I still can."

At this point in a Hollywood film a fatherly embodiment of wisdom like Jimmy Stewart would have materialized and explained how, and why, Danny's quest after "the good life" was misguided at best and was at worst hurtful to his family. Beginning, of course, with the rather obvious observation that there wasn't anything he had done in the last six months that could remotely be construed as part of a good life. And the apparent pinnacle in his telling—throwing cash at casino employees—didn't seem so ideal.

I didn't have the age or the experience or the confidence that such paternalism would have required. Besides, we were both tired. So I let the moment pass.

Still, Danny seemed subdued and thoughtful. As if, maybe, he had begun to think about his life in a slightly different way. Perhaps what I mistook for thoughtfulness was no more than the fatigue of a late night. And so I left him, still leaning on the bedside table, as he had been when I came in, but now with an empty glass. I suggested he might want to rinse the glass out and hide the bottle before the charge nurse came in. *He* really *was* an asshole. Danny didn't say anything, just smiled and waved. I saluted—it seemed appropriate, somehow.

I suppose I remember Danny's story clearly, at least in part, because he behaved so badly. But I also remember Danny's story because parts of it don't fit together. Of course, Danny did want to play the role of the big man in town, for a while. That is, his boorish behavior was motivated by exactly the reason he gave me that night. He was a man who, stung by some ill-defined and misdirected sense of missed opportunity, methodically began to drink, gamble, and to inflate his sense of his own importance. Although not particularly admirable, his was a harmless-enough goal, or it would have been, if Danny hadn't raided his family's checking account in order to pursue it.

But his story was much more complex. There was, I think, an element of distraction that drove Danny to the bars, and which goaded him to prepare for his hospitalization by adding a bottle of Scotch to his overnight bag. Too, he was trying to reach back to some of the experiences he'd had as a young man. And it was also a celebration, of a sort. So, as I've gotten some distance from the conversation Danny and I had that night, I find I've grown sympathetic to, if not quite supportive of, whatever goals had motivated him to act the way he did.

When I first sat down on the bed across from him, Danny had looked depleted, reduced. But taking a last look at him on my way out the door that morning, I had the impression of someone who wasn't diminished so much as incomplete and unfinished, as if he were waiting for a sculptor to make a couple of well-placed strikes with a chisel. He was almost done, but needed a little more work.

I didn't see Danny the next day. He went for his procedure late, and I'd left for the day by the time he got out. The Iowa City grapevine being what it was, though, I was able to keep tabs on Danny from a distance, like a field biologist tracking a particularly ornery and antisocial grizzly bear by examining the debris he left in his wake.

From what I could tell, Danny did not turn over a new leaf, but he did become much more careful about his money. For instance, he stopped gambling, or so I heard. And I also heard that he was no longer the source of free drinks that he had always been. A disappointment, I'm sure, to the other bar patrons, but also a relief, I imagine, to his family. And about six months later I heard that he had died at home with hospice, cared for by his wife.

THREE

Alberto

Reconnection and Reconciliation

Alberto

Alberto might have died without receiving any medical care at all if it weren't for a medical resident in my program who, fortunately, was a loyal patron of the bars of Iowa City. Late one December evening, apparently, the staff at one popular establishment found Alberto asleep on a wooden bench against the back wall when they made the rounds for last call. No one was sure how long he had been there.

They tried to wake Alberto, without success. I don't know what methods they used, but I'm sure they knew their business. They were stunned, I'm sure, by their failure, which was probably a rare and humbling event. Yet they were prevented by Iowa's high standards of civility from dumping him on the icy sidewalk. So the bartender called the police to take Alberto to the city jail, where he would at least be safe for the night.

But my colleague, who is nothing if not conscientious, was also still there at closing time. And he was the one who noticed, as the police lifted Alberto to carry him to the squad car, that the right side of Alberto's face was sagging. So he suggested to the police that Alberto might actually be sick—my colleague suggested a stroke—and that an ambulance might be more appropriate than a police van.

I'm sure that in situations like this the police get all sorts of unsolicited advice, much of it useless. Indeed, if I were in their shoes, I would have been skeptical of the unsolicited advice of someone claiming to be a doctor but who was in a bar at closing time on a Wednesday night. My colleague is a superb physician, but that is not the sort of setting that inspires confidence.

In any event, my colleague prevailed and the ambulance crew, when they arrived, was able to confirm that Alberto did in fact have a complete right-sided paralysis. So they took him to our emergency room, where a CT scan revealed a large mass on the left side of Alberto's brain, dramatic enough to be clearly visible even to the medical student on our team. We weren't sure what the mass was, so he was admitted for an evaluation.

When I first saw Alberto, he was lying on a gurney just outside the CT suite in the hospital's basement. He was short but solid, with incongruously short arms and a barrel chest. Even supine and inert he seemed to have a surprising density and hardness, like a dried kidney bean. He had a round, pockmarked face, coated by a sheen of oil and sweat and wrapped in several days of stubble that had crept unevenly up and over his cheekbones like a rough sort of lichen. And he seemed to be only half-conscious. His right eye was closed completely, and his left came to life sleepily for a few moments at a time and then eased shut.

As I stood at the foot of Alberto's gurney, the corridor's flickering lemonade-yellow fluorescent light washed over both of us, giving our late-night meeting an illicit feel. I had an uneasy foreboding, as though we'd been caught by a security camera. And that sense was mirrored in my own thinking about possible causes of Alberto's condition, all of which were either bad (an infection) or very bad (a tumor). Particularly if the mass turned out to be a malignant tumor, there would be very little treatment that we could offer him.

But as I reached this grim conclusion I realized that Alberto was awake and watching me with his good left eye. And not just watching me—he was grinning. A big, silly—albeit lopsided—grin. Without warning, he stuck his left arm in my general direction, meaty thumb up, waving it uncertainly but vigorously, like an enthusiastic but demented lobster.

It was, I realized, an offer of a handshake. The best he could do, it was barely recognizable, but still irresistible. I took his left hand in mine clumsily in what turned into the odd but functional grip you'd use, say, for thumb wrestling.

"*¡Hola! ¿Cómo estás? Yo soy Alberto. ¿Cómo te llamas?*" Alberto's words were slurred and my Spanish was rusty. As I was working on a suitable response to this salvo, I realized that Alberto was fast asleep again. A rather harsh commentary on my conversational skills, I thought. But at least it was a start. I made my way back upstairs to the ward, still uncertain about what we could offer him, but more optimistic, too. At least there would be Spanish lessons to look forward to. And thumb wrestling.

Over the next few days a series of rushed tests and a biopsy confirmed that the mass in Alberto's brain was a glioblastoma—about the worst possible diagnosis—and we guessed that he had about two months to live. This was awful news, of course, but we knew that a large dose of steroids could decrease the tumor's swelling and help him to feel dramatically better, at least for a few weeks. And indeed, three days later Alberto was more awake, and after a few more days he was strong enough for a shave and a bath. Soon his face, still lopsided, would crease into an enormous comma whenever he smiled, which was almost constantly. His right-sided wink of a smile would occasionally flash a single gold tooth, as if he were shyly displaying a prized possession.

As his condition improved, he soon tired of replaying our first, left-handed handshake. Instead, he began to use his left hand to pick up his right arm, holding it out like a marionette's limb, with even greater enthusiasm. He also recovered enough to give the social worker his Social Security number, which he remembered after some difficulty, so the hospital could bill Medicaid.

And he recovered enough to talk incessantly, with a breathless enthusiasm, about his family. As he did, he'd spill details about them in a rambling, haphazard way. He told us that his father had died years before, for instance. And that it had been his father's death that led him to move north from Guatemala so he could work to support his family. We also learned that he had two younger twin brothers, nineteen years old, who were wild kids, *"locos."* They weren't much help to their mother—always fixing up their cars and never helping. But they were good kids. And his little sister—here he smiled again—she was a diamond, going to be a doctor or a lawyer. And of course his mother: long-suffering, with a heart of gold.

What emerged most clearly from these rambling monologues was that Alberto wanted more than anything to see his family again. That, he said, was *"la más importante,"* the most important. He would ask us, repeatedly, to find them. That was all he wanted, he said. He'd become agitated, then, reaching out with his good arm and asking one of us—whoever was closest—to take his hand. As if whatever promises we made to find his family would be more enforceable, and therefore more believable, if they were sealed by the solemn pressure of that grip.

But Alberto's feverish enthusiasm about his family did little to disguise the fact that he couldn't do anything to help us find them. He could paint pictures of them that were vivid enough to render them unmistakable if we happened to meet them on the streets of Iowa City. But he couldn't give us a single clue that we could use to track them down. No addresses or phone numbers, for instance, and not even the name of the city where they lived. It was as if, by telling us details about his family, he was certain that we would be that much more energetic in searching for them. As if that energy, without any information, would be enough.

What we didn't say, but which Alberto almost certainly knew, was that we didn't have much time. At some point soon, the steroids we were giving him to control the swelling in his brain would not be able to keep up with the tumor's growth. We'd need to think then about other measures, like a shunt that would relieve some of the pressure inside his skull. But even a shunt would help only temporarily, and Alberto would rapidly lose what little cognitive and physical function we'd been able to preserve. So if he wanted us to find his family, and if he hoped to be awake enough to recognize them when they arrived, we guessed that we had a week or two at most.

The Need for Connection

A final connection with friends and family has become a defining feature of the way most of us would like our lives to end. Indeed, these sorts of connections are the most visible, and most memorable, aspects of the ways in which people die. These connections are so moving, and so memorable, in fact, that I've used them as highlights of lectures to medical students and nursing students about what their patients might imagine a good death would look like.

I'm a researcher, and so it's natural in these lectures for me to describe studies of the way that people think of a good death. And almost all of these studies underscore the importance to patients of renewing or restoring connections with friends and families. In fact, in the first study of this topic these connections proved to be one of the most important aspects of dying well, and other subsequent studies have found the same thing. But I'm often dismayed to find that, for these data-fatigued students who are tired of numbers and facts, studies often seem to have less impact than stories do.

So I might tell them instead about Larry Heath, a death-row inmate in Alabama who chose to forgo his last meal in order to spend an additional thirty minutes with his wife and family. Or I might tell them about one of many tragic telephone calls on September 11, 2001, to family members, like that between Tom

McGinnis, trapped on the ninety-second floor of the North Tower of the World Trade Center, and his wife, Iliana, as they shared a few final words before the telephone line went dead.

Or sometimes, if I'm not confident that these examples have captured their imagination, I reach for a more epic tale. At the height of London's Great Plague in 1665–66, the enveloping fear of being taken ill prompted Londoners to make intricate contingency plans. For instance, Samuel Pepys, who was perhaps the best-known chronicler of that period, describes a heated battle within his family about where his sister should live during the worst months. Pepys wanted to send her to Huntingdonshire, a rural district just west of Cambridge that is now an hour's drive due north of London on the A1, thinking that she would be safest there. But her husband, Anthony, selfishly wanted her closer, in Windsor, so that they could be together if he should become ill.

In fact, it was so common for people to travel to be near loved ones as they were dying that district aldermen published notices identifying these travelers so that they could be caught and quarantined. And funerals were banned altogether for the same reason. Eventually, Edward Hyde, the Earl of Clarendon, directed that magistrates should use "all force & rigour" to prevent funerals, and the Lord Mayor of London, Sir John Lawrence, directed his aldermen to stop them.

Understanding a Desire for Connection

I use these examples in lectures and during bedside rounds to emphasize the importance of connections with family, but I admit they do little to explain people's motivations. What is it that drives those of us who are near the end of life, as Alberto was, to renew or restore connections with friends and family? Why at this point, but not sooner?

There is a fascinating line of research that has begun to answer this question, albeit indirectly. Laura Carstensen is a psychologist who has studied how we perceive time and how our perceptions of time affect the decisions we make. In particular, one line of her research has evaluated situations in which—either naturally or by the design of an experiment—people believe that their time is limited. Over the course of several studies, Carstensen has been able to examine how this perception of limited time influences our decisions.

Although these experiments are difficult to reduce to simple explanations, it appears that when our time is limited—or at least when we perceive it to be—we tend to focus our attention on relationships. Perhaps the study that showed this result most clearly was one in which Carstensen interviewed three groups of people, with three distinct life expectancies: healthy adults, adults with asymptomatic HIV infection, and adults with more advanced HIV. Carstensen asked study subjects in each group to make choices about the kinds of people they would prefer to spend time with.

She found that whereas the healthy adults were more likely to choose to spend time with someone who is interesting, such as the author of a book they had just read, those who were HIV positive were more likely to choose someone with whom they have shared interests or experiences. That is, they would choose people who might become friends. This was particularly true for those people who were HIV positive and had a significantly diminished life expectancy. Interestingly, Carstensen has also found that older people, whose life expectancy is limited by age rather than by illness, make similar choices to HIV patients and place a greater value on the emotional content of potential relationships.

Therefore, people whose life expectancy is limited by illness or age do seem to be predisposed (and some would say even hardwired) to connect with others. I find that there is a certain appeal to the simplicity of these sorts of explanations. Indeed, they offer a clear motivation that has the elemental force of a reflex.

But an increasing focus on relationships is not simply a goal in and of itself. Instead, these sorts of reconnections with family members constitute the foundation for other choices that people make.

For instance, if Alberto had wanted to craft a final message that would define the way people would remember him, it would almost certainly be his family to whom that message would be directed. Or if he felt that he owed anyone an apology before he died, again, it would probably be to his family. And if he had in mind a final celebration, who better than his two crazy younger brothers to join him? And so, all psychology aside, one motivation for reconnecting with family is that these reconnections give a foundation—and often an audience—for all that we hope to do in whatever time we have left.

Perhaps this explains why many of my seriously ill patients choose to focus their time and attention on a few close relationships. When I mentioned this phenomenon once to a friend who is a structural engineer, he told me about a principle of engineering known as Barba's Law. This rule, as I understand it, predicts that structures subjected to stress will fracture along predicable lines. In families subjected to the stresses of a terminal illness, I often see the same thing. No matter how large a patient's circle of friends and families may be, that network of relationships often undergoes a sort of controlled disintegration, leaving only those that are most important.

Whether it's intentional or not, an intensified focus on close relationships has an important functional role. It is these close relationships—with people who know us best—that are most likely to provide the support and advice that we need in making decisions about health care. At least these are the people that we tend to rely on, and are generally the people we want close by to make decisions for us if we become unable to.

And as people with serious illnesses near the end of life, they begin to rely increasingly on others to share health care decisions with them. As a patient's health deteriorates, new medical problems create cognitive impairment and stir up symptoms like pain or fatigue that make it difficult to concentrate on making health care decisions. At the same time, those decisions become more challenging. And so as the complexity of these decisions outstrips patients' ability to understand and process information, they draw on family members for help. We've found, for instance, that this shift can be accelerated by depression, which is common in serious illness. We've also found that by the time patients with serious illness are ready to enroll in hospice—usually in the last months of life—their families are almost always involved in the decision.

I should note that there is a danger here of what philosophers call the "naturalistic fallacy," that is, of confusing what happens with what ought to happen. Simply because many people focus their attention on a small number of close relationships doesn't mean that they should. In fact, many of my patients create new relationships and find them to be meaningful and rewarding. Still, as my patients near the end of life, and as they face diminishing time and energy, they must make increasingly difficult choices about how to spend their time, and with whom. And it seems to me that the result is often an intensifying of those relationships that have always been most important.

Overcoming Barriers

When I talk to medical students about the importance of relationships and connections near the end of life, I realize that even the best studies can't hold the students' attention with the grip that Alberto's story does. What makes his story so compelling for them is not simply his desire to see his family, but rather all the obstacles that were placed in his way. It's those obstacles that make for an engaging narrative, and it was this narrative, in turn, that rallied us around him and encouraged us to help find his family.

Alberto's story shows more vividly than most that although it is so important for us to strengthen our relationships with others, doing so can also be enormously difficult. There are, of course, the pressures of the circumstances. Serious illness brings severe symptoms, not the least of which can be incapacitating fatigue. In addition, the late stages of serious illness are often accompanied by a loss of cognitive ability that is either temporary or permanent. The result, all too often, is a series of dense barriers that separate patients from their friends and family.

These are the sorts of barriers that are obvious, and which we try to correct whenever possible. For instance, in the last days or weeks of life many patients—perhaps as many as 30 percent—will develop delirium, which is a syndrome of confusion and disorientation that is often accompanied by visual hallucinations. Delirium can be frightening to patients who experience it, and to family members who observe it. But the most important consequence of delirium is often the barrier that it creates between patients and their families, robbing them of a final opportunity to spend time together. And so we often use medications both to quiet the visible, "active" symptoms of delirium, and to try to restore a level of consciousness that would allow meaningful interaction.

If we're successful, our efforts to treat delirium under these circumstances offer us a potent dose of satisfaction. It's a chance, sometimes, to see patients wake up enough to spend meaningful time with their families. When that happens, it feels as though we've added a few hours or days to the patient's life. Unfortunately, though, not all barriers to a final connection are so easily overcome.

Constraint and Distance

I took care of a retired English professor once who was dying of an indolent but relentless form of leukemia. That George's death wasn't imminent was, I suppose, a blessing. But because of a cruel but common trick that some cancers play, the nature of his leukemia also meant that there were no treatments that could affect its course. That is, like other slow-growing malignancies, George's was particularly resistant to chemotherapy. And for George, any promise that his death wouldn't come soon was outweighed by certainty that there was nothing at all that he could do to delay it.

During the two years since his diagnosis, his wife told me, he had become increasingly distant—and occasionally antagonistic—to friends and family. He would refuse dinner invitations without a plausible explanation, for instance, and he would avoid large gatherings of people. Even when they had guests visiting, he would often retreat to his study, closing the door behind him.

His oncologist was initially concerned, and asked George to see a psychiatrist, who didn't prove to be particularly helpful. The psychiatrist was reasonably certain, however, that George wasn't depressed. This was a relief to the oncologist, perhaps, but didn't do much to reassure George's wife. I met George when he was hospitalized briefly for pneumonia, and she'd taken me aside for a chat as the intern examined George just before he and I were introduced. During a hurried conference outside, she told me that she was still worried about George's behavior.

She'd seemed so worried, in fact, that later on that evening, after she had gone home, I asked George how things had been going for him. But he was noncommittal. "Fine," he said. Things had been fine.

It was a peculiar change in his demeanor. For the past twenty minutes or so, our interaction had been a back-and-forth bantering in which George was always one step ahead of me. It had a rhythm that was not too different, perhaps, than the rhythm his conversations with his students had taken on years before. He'd even been lighthearted and jocular as we talked about the reason he was in the hospital. (George: A lot of famous people die of pneumonia, don't they? Me: I didn't know you were famous. George: I would be if I died.) He'd told me, too, about a secret trout stream in northern Iowa and had promised to give me directions. And yet, suddenly, a simple question about his well-being made him strangely standoffish. And so I asked him about the sudden change.

He didn't want people's sympathy, he told me. It just seemed so . . . unnatural, and forced. As if people were struggling to be kind and considerate. As if they were following a script they had to read.

No, he continued, thinking. That wasn't really it. It was more that their concern created a barrier between him and everyone else. Even if that concern was carefully expressed and well meaning— especially then—George felt as though that concern separated him from everyone else.

He was particularly irritated, he told me, when people twisted their conversation in an ungainly limbo to avoid speaking about the future. He told me about how one conversation in which his long-time friends were gingerly evading talk of the next presidential election brought tears of anger, and also of gratitude. Gratitude that his friends would be so thoughtful, but also anger that their consideration had reminded him that he would not live to see the next election. I realized that my consideration, like his friends', which was meant to close the distance between us, paradoxically created a barrier by emphasizing that our futures—mine and his—were diverging.

It was, he said, like being confined with death in a small closet. Or a carriage. He smiled—for the first time since my awkward question rearranged out relationship—and looked at me curiously, one eyebrow raised. There was some allusion that I was missing, but what?

He shook his head in mock sadness. Wasn't I familiar with Emily Dickinson, he asked me? But he didn't wait; my dumb expression was all the answer he needed. As he recited a few lines for me, his loping mellow baritone reminded me that he had been one of the university's most popular professors.

> *Because I could not stop for Death—*
> *He kindly stopped for me—*
> *The Carriage held but just Ourselves—*
> *And Immortality.*

Existing as a dying person was bad enough, he explained, forced into the habit of anticipating death and editing one's future. But the real difficulty, the real challenge, was created by bystanders. To them, the dying person is already dead, or almost. They are made sympathetic and cautious by the person's illness. Even worse, they become uncomfortable, and embarrassed by their own health. And—his main point—their discomfort is isolating. The dying person becomes an object of sympathy. And that sympathy, however well-meaning, confines the dying person in a carriage with only his death for company, and sends him on his way.

As I listened, I heard a persuasive justification of his own behavior. But it was a justification that was practiced and polished. And it was delivered not in the hesitant, hopeful way that a patient might explain his behavior to his physician, but rather as a carefully crafted lesson. We might well have been in a lecture hall that evening.

His delivery was so smooth, in fact, that it wasn't until several days later, when I had found Dickinson's poem at a local bookstore, that I realized that George's entire lesson had been in the third person. "One feels trapped," he'd said. "One feels the rest of the world pulling away." And only now do I recognize that the course along which George steered his sentences, through neutral grammatical territory, was a way of heading off any expression from me of the sympathy that he abhorred.

Even now, armed with that insight and additional years of experience, I'm not sure what I could have done to help George that night. He was right, I've come to realize, that sympathy and consideration are—or can be—isolating. So I left him that night no better off than I found him, except with a plan for treating his pneumonia that would send him back home in a day or two.

But perhaps because I identified with his situation, and because I could see myself in his shoes someday, I tried to imagine a solution for him. And that solution eventually took the form of a novel. It was about a steady, pedantic geography professor, recently divorced, coasting into his sixties. An indifferent scholar and a failure as a father and husband, he is, oddly, an outstanding teacher. In fact, his talents in the lecture hall have won him numerous awards from his students and even puzzled admiration from his colleagues. When he is diagnosed with prostate cancer, he becomes oppressed by the syrupy solicitousness of his colleagues, his ex-wife, and his children. He responds by treating his cancer with humor, which prompts worried whispers about his mental health and inflames the sympathy that he found so annoying. When he comes home one evening to find that some well-meaning soul has delivered a week's worth of reheatable meals, he snaps. He quits his job, closes up his house, and disappears.

He turns up at the cancer clinic of a large city where he knows no one. Starting fresh, he masquerades as a retired tour guide, a ruse that his knowledge of geography makes entirely plausible. He is happily anonymous, and his relationship with his doctors and nurses is purely businesslike. He finds a furnished studio apartment near the hospital where he is by several decades the oldest resident. He falls into his old role of teacher and counselor and even succeeds in passing as healthy for a time, until his secret leaks out. The members of his newly adopted family in his building are predictably solicitous—oppressively so, at least at first—but this iteration turns out better. Now the professor is in a better position to retreat when he needs to. But he can also accept their help and sympathy, and slowly, he does.

The problem, of course, is that I got rather attached to the professor and didn't want to see him die. Particularly since I had William Hurt in mind for the movie version of my novel, and I'd read somewhere that Hurt refuses to be in a movie in which he dies. True or not, it wasn't a chance I wanted to take. So I left the professor and ultimately the book in limbo.

Although the novel was never finished, sketching the story did give me a better sense of what George might have been feeling. My fictional solution—an escape to a new city and a new identity—is obviously not one that I could have suggested to George that night. But I do think that it's one that he would have found appealing.

Or perhaps George didn't need an escape so much as he needed a respite. Perhaps new relationships with people who didn't think of him as "dying" would have given him the respite that he needed. So I wonder if there was, in fact, a solution in the escape I created for his fictional character. For instance, there might have been a way that George could have excluded his illness from some relationships entirely, without moving to another city. Instead, I imagined, George might simply have made a handful of new friends who didn't know about his illness.

In fact, even smaller changes might have reduced the solicitude that George found so difficult to bear. One of my oncologist colleagues routinely suggests to his patients that they take special care of themselves and their appearance. He does this, he tells me, mostly to give his patients confidence. But he also thinks that doing so puts others at ease and helps them to forget, at least temporarily, about the patient's illness.

Or maybe George could have used humor to push back against the sympathy that he perceived, forcing his way through the barriers that it created. A lighthearted joking about illness and death can put some people off at first, but often puts them at ease eventually. I saw this transformation most clearly in a patient I took care of once who had a form of leukemia that was similar to George's and who, coincidentally, was also a teacher. She was young—in her thirties—a sad fact that produced in all of us a sort of pious gloom. Her immediate and extended family, when they came to visit her, were also melancholy, almost funereal.

That premature mourning made her furious. She found it stifling. She wanted to spend whatever time she had left interacting with her family as the person that she was, not as the dying person everyone seemed to see.

So she fought back. When anyone asked her how she was doing she would say, brightly, "I'm not dead yet," or "I'm dying, how are you?" This carefully calibrated note of flippancy flustered the medical student taking care of her, and it also concerned her husband and her mother, at least at first. "How could she be joking at a time like this?" they wanted to know. Their concern prompted a great deal of discussion among us, which in turn led to a psychiatry consult.

But soon we all realized that this was her way of putting us at ease, and making explicit what we were all thinking. I say that we realized this as if this were a puzzle that we eventually solved, but that's not really true. It was more as if she was teaching us. More than that, I think she was using us—her doctors and nurses—as an example. She understood that humor could dissolve the barrier that separated her from her family, and she was teaching us so that we could help her family understand that her humor was healthy. She would joke with us about her medications, tests, procedures, and especially about her prognosis ("So, let me get this straight—when the mail comes, I should toss the bills and open those credit card offers instead?"). And she was at her funniest, and most vibrant, when her family was in the room.

And just as she had planned, we learned to joke with her. Her family was understandably awkward, at first. But we explained, as best we could, what we thought was going on. Fortified by our interpretation, and prompted by our example, her family gradually became more comfortable in their interactions with her. In effect, we had given them permission to act more naturally, to play the roles that she had in mind for them. Their visits became more instinctive, less tightly choreographed, and closer, I think, to what she had hoped for.

I think that this approach, or something like it, would have been ideal for George. And he could have pulled it off, easily. He was certainly intelligent and funny enough. Moreover, his years spent teaching—an occupation that is only one step removed from acting—would have equipped him well. This was a strategy that I might have suggested that night. If I saw George today, though, I would probably simply do my best to help him share his concerns with his family. I'd help him to explain to them what he described so eloquently to me, with the same humor and the same light touch.

But I like to think that I wouldn't need to. In fact, I like to think that George arrived at much the same solution on his own and that perhaps his explanation that night was a rehearsal for what he would say—without my help—to his friends and family.

Protecting Others

Sometimes the barriers to connection that we face are those that we create for ourselves. I'm thinking in particular of the way that some of my patients distance themselves from friends and family members, and particularly from children, in an effort to lessen the impact of loss. Although this is something that I've seen in many of my patients, the best example I can think of comes from a very different source.

I was flying to New York—oddly enough, to meet with several publishers to pitch the idea of this book—when my flight from Phoenix was canceled. During an increasingly frantic phone call with one of the airline's ticket agents, in order to convey just how important it was that I be in New York the following morning, I told the woman about the reason for my trip and about the book. Although I was not particularly coherent, the idea seemed to register with her. (It was, I thought, a good omen). And as she found me another flight, she told me about her mother, who had pancreatic cancer that was advanced when it was diagnosed.

In the months leading up to the diagnosis, her mother had been growing weak and losing weight. And her decline seemed to accelerate rapidly after the diagnosis was made, as if naming the trouble somehow gave the cancer strength. Throughout what was only a few months between her diagnosis and death, her mother spent more time with the ticket agent's daughters, her only grandchildren. She would take them shopping, on "lunch dates," and, once, on a limousine ride around town.

But she never, as far as the agent knew, told her granddaughters about her illness. Up until the last weeks of her life, when she became too weak to leave the house and they eventually recognized her condition, she was adamant that her granddaughters shouldn't know. She didn't want them to be sad, she said. And she wanted above all for the time they spent together to be happy.

And so the agent's mother would carefully stage-manage her visits and the events she planned. She would devote meticulous care to her makeup and clothes to hide as much as possible her pallor and wasted body. She would arrange a taxi to pick them up and ferry them around. And, Cinderella-like, she would ensure that the entire outing was no more than two hours, which was all she had the strength to endure.

On one hand, she felt the need to connect with her granddaughters, spending time with them, and ensuring that they would remember her. On the other hand, she was aware that their time together would be painful for them if they knew that she was dying. And so she created a delicate drama that offered a sense of connection, keeping within strict limits.

I don't mean to imply that this example illustrates some ideal solution. Far from it. In fact, one could argue that the ticket agent's mother deprived her granddaughters of a valuable experience. Those outings might have been much more meaningful if the girls had known that their grandmother was dying. Perhaps they would have paid closer attention, experienced that time together more fully, and remembered those trips more vividly. So her granddaughters lost something valuable as a result of their grandmother's protectiveness (aided, of course, by their mother's collusion).

I love this story not because it was exemplary, but because the ticket agent I spoke with remembered it that way. Where I saw a woman who was afraid to be honest with her family—and afraid, perhaps, of what emotions might be let loose—the agent saw a woman who was fiercely brave. She saw a woman who, even in the last weeks of her life, thought only about what was best for her granddaughters.

The ticket agent's mother is hardly unique. I think this desire to protect others motivates many of my patients. And I usually find myself torn between two conflicting interpretations. On one hand, this need to shield others from the pain of loss, or even the knowledge of illness, seems misguided. Certainly, it creates barriers and distance between close friends and family members at a point in time when relationships are most important. This is, more or less, the "standard" interpretation that most of us who work in the area of end-of-life care would hold, that the desire to protect others creates a barrier to strengthening relationships near the end of life. And that this is a barrier we should help our patients and their families to overcome.

On the other hand, I also find that I have a sneaking sympathy for those who forgo the proximity and support of others in order to protect them. That they need not—most of the time—forgo these relationships is beside the point. Simply the fact that people are willing to act in this way seems to me to be a wonderful testament to human nature.

Still, this was probably not the best outcome. If I'd been taking care of that ticket agent's mother, I would have tried to understand why she felt so strongly that she needed to protect her granddaughters from the knowledge of her illness. And I would have tried to help her to determine for herself whether the benefits of the protection she offered them really outweighed the more meaningful interactions that her granddaughters were missing. Perhaps, together, we might even have created a compromise that gave the girls a sense of the significance of these outings that they would appreciate and remember.

Lack of a Script

For many of us, the most daunting challenge to reestablishing connections and strengthening relationships is the lack of guide—a script—for what to do and what to say. In fact, many people who die of serious illnesses are left on their own to choreograph their last conversations and connections with friends and families. In that regard, I sometimes think that we're not much better off than trapped miners dying alone in the darkness of a low-ceilinged tunnel, trying to scratch a few words on a scrap of paper.

A few of my colleagues see this as an opportunity. Ira Byock is perhaps the best example. Ira is a friend and colleague who has written a series of books for the general public that are designed to provide patients and families with a script, or at least a template, of what to say. Although these sorts of books risk being preachy or rigid, Ira's are neither. He succeeds in providing both a structure and, more important, ideas and options.

But I think the opportunities are broader than this. Certainly, there's a great deal that we can all learn from books like Ira's, and we should. But we can also learn from each other. Actually, Ira and I would probably both agree that his books are so useful as guides because they come from lessons that he's learned from his own patients.

And just as we've learned from our patients, occasionally, my patients learn from each other. I once took care of a man with esophageal cancer who was having increasing difficulty swallowing. Soon Arnold wouldn't be able to swallow at all, and he needed to decide whether to undergo surgery. He wanted his family to be aware of his decision, so one afternoon they all gathered in the multipurpose room down the hall from Arnold's room. He'd included his wife, of course, and a granddaughter who was in nursing school nearby, and seven or eight other family members I'd never met.

The intern and I described the surgical procedure and laid out its risks, which were considerable, as well as its potential benefits, which were uncertain. I knew from our previous conversations that Arnold wanted to avoid surgery, and so the unfavorable picture that the intern and I painted that afternoon was a bit of amateur theater, emphasizing the negative in hopes that Arnold's family would understand and support his choice. Arnold seemed to consider his options carefully and, warming to the role of the ambivalent patient, even asked a few questions. Finally, though, he said he really didn't see what surgery would accomplish, and that he'd rather not go through it. There was some discussion, but, as we had anticipated, not much. We made alternative plans—dietary changes, alterations to his medications to make them easier to swallow—and then the meeting ended.

Just as we were getting up to leave, though, Arnold surprised everyone when he asked us all to stay for a moment. The intern and I stood uncertainly for a moment in the doorway. But Arnold waved to us, asking us to come back, and we slipped into the chairs we had just left.

Arnold took a pair of reading glasses from the chest pocket of his hospital pajamas, adjusting them on the tip of his nose. It was an odd transformation—I had never seen this retired farmer with glasses—that left him looking suddenly professorial. Then he pulled a sheet of note paper from under the blanket in his lap, folded lengthwise half a dozen times, accordionlike. He gripped the outer edges tightly between gnarled thumb and forefinger, flattening the creases as best he could, and began to read.

The text was brief, no more than a long paragraph. He was lucky to have such a wonderful family, he began. He wished that he had spent more time with each of them (and here he read out their names and a few words about each of them). And he didn't want surgery, and a hospital stay, to take away even more time. There were other things, but that's what I remember most clearly.

His family was tearful, and pleased, but most of all they were surprised. Arnold was generally quiet and undemonstrative. Gentle but passive, and usually untroubled by strong opinions except, occasionally, about the University of Iowa football team. His granddaughter looked at me, suspecting that I had orchestrated this.

I hadn't, but I knew who had. A few days before the family meeting, I had been talking with Arnold in his room when another patient was using their shared telephone. (At that time, our VA hospital had four beds to a room, and each room's telephone was placed next to the door.) Arnold and I could hear only one side of the conversation, but I gleaned enough to guess that the man was talking to someone in another hospital. Arnold told me later that the man's brother was going into surgery for replacement of a heart valve, which posed a significant risk given his previous surgery. I didn't know that then but suspected, nevertheless, that this was a serious and perhaps final conversation.

The curtain around Arnold's bed was pulled—a farcical convention that health care providers employ to convince ourselves that we're offering our patients some sort of privacy—and so his roommate was a disembodied voice. I noticed that the cadence of his speech was oddly fast, almost high-pitched. Not abnormally so, but enough to make me wonder what he did for a living. He sounded young, and I guessed he was in some form of business. He sounded like he was used to selling something, convincing people. (It turned out, according to Arnold, that he was retired, but had been an English teacher all his life).

I felt uncomfortable eavesdropping, and it was becoming obvious that Arnold wasn't paying attention to our own discussion of the risks and benefits of a feeding tube to bypass the narrowing in his esophagus. And, honestly, neither was I. Given the conversation going on not five feet from us, a discussion of bloating and diarrhea seemed inappropriate if not disrespectful. So I said I would be back later to finish our discussion.

As I left, I slid past the patient on the telephone, parked in his wheelchair just inside the door. He leaned over just enough to let me pass, not rudely, but as if he were absorbed in his conversation. As I sidled through the doorway, I heard one phrase that I remembered clearly, telling his brother how lucky he had been to have such a wonderful family.

I love this story because it serves as a reminder that my patients can look to a variety of sources for guidance. They can and, I think, they should. The challenge of finding the right thing to say is so daunting that I want very much to think that we can learn from each others' messages. A form of eavesdropping can expand our own vision of what's possible, and what we could say.

Imagine that you have to leave a message for your family right now. And imagine that you have a minute, or maybe two, to say whatever you need to. Would you say the right thing? That is, would you say everything you wanted to say, in the way you wanted to say it? It's hard to imagine that any of us would.

But what if you had a chance to overhear other conversations? What if you could take at least some of those words and craft your own message? That message would still be yours, but it would be better informed, better prepared.

Arnold was able to use some of the language that he and I overheard. But what is perhaps more important, he also used his roommate's example. And sometimes all that is needed is an example—an idea—of what's possible. That was the case when a small group of sailors survived the sinking of the *Hornet*, a clipper ship bound for San Francisco, and found themselves in an impossibly small lifeboat in the middle of the Pacific. Their captain, Josiah Mitchell, became their example, writing a last message to his family. Others, inspired, asked for paper. And so Mitchell passed around paper, and they agreed that the last man remaining alive should lash the bottle with all of their messages in it to the lifeboat. (We know about this drama, and Mitchell's role in it, because he and a few others survived to tell their story, launching the career, incidentally, of the young reporter Samuel Clemens, better known as Mark Twain.)

But very few of us will have examples like that of Mitchell, or Arnold's roommate, which is why these sorts of connections are a priority for hospice programs. For instance, hospice social workers or bereavement counselors often organize what is called a "life review," which organizes memories—through pictures and stories and artifacts—in a cohesive way. The primary purpose of a life review is to provide a sense of closure and to leave a legacy to family. But the process of collecting pictures and telling stories requires, or at least facilitates, conversations among family members. So a life review often provides a script that builds connections.

And other health care providers also have a role to play. The nurse practitioner I work with, Pat Chriss, is wonderfully adept at suggesting elements of a script. She doesn't plan a conversation, nor does she try to stage-manage one. Instead, she asks our patients and their families to think about what they would like to say to each other. What would you want your daughter to know, she asks them? And what would you want your father to tell you? These questions are nondirective and flexible, less elements of a script, even, than they are building blocks for a connection.

When I have these conversations, though, I also try to make sure my patients understand that the words they use may not be nearly as important as the effort that they make. Consider, for instance, what it must have been like for Arnold's family to share that moment with him. What they appreciated most and, probably, what they will remember best, is not so much the words that Arnold read so unevenly from that sheet of notepaper. Instead, it seems to me that it was Arnold's effort to have that conversation, and the thought and preparation he devoted to it, that were most meaningful. That, to me, is the real message.

Forms of Connections

Many of my colleagues seem to be guided by rather firm and fixed ideas about the way that patients should make connections as they near the end of life. Some insist, for instance, on involving as many members of a patient's family as possible. Others emphasize apologies and forgiveness. These prescriptions can be so idiosyncratic, in fact, that I often find myself wondering about the past experiences that have led a particular colleague to his or her own ideal.

But over time I've become open to a wide variety of last conversations. And I've come to appreciate, too, that the actual connections that take place often extend far below the surface of what we, as health care providers, can see. I learned this lesson not from one of my patients, but from a fascinating series of portraits, many of which are on display at the Kunsthaus, the main art museum in Zurich.

Ferdinand Hodler was a Swiss Art Nouveau painter in the late nineteenth and early twentieth centuries whose mistress, Valentine Godé-Darel, was diagnosed with cancer in 1914. From her diagnosis to her death about a year later, Hodler created a series of paintings and sketches that documented her gradual decline. In the first paintings, Godé-Darel maintains an upright pose, her gaze fixed on the viewer. In these portraits she is well dressed, even prim. We see her head and shoulders only, perfectly symmetrical, with black hair tightly framing a narrow, angular face. That image is direct, immediate, and, while not really warm or inviting, at least directly engaging.

Over the succeeding months, though, she is transformed, slowly and agonizingly. We see her next in her bed, leaning against pillows that lend support to her thin neck, with the rest of her emaciated body in the frame. That change alone seems to make her much more vulnerable. Gradually, she slips down, reaching an angle of repose that is almost, but not quite, supine. In that transition her gaze shifts as well. We no longer feel her gaze or even see her eyes clearly. She begins to turn her attention elsewhere, away from the viewer and, one suspects, away from Hodler as well. The result, by the end, is a slow transformation from Hodler's mistress who looks out at us directly to an anonymous woman who is a passive object.

Walking slowly through the museum's galleries, viewing some of these portraits mixed with Hodler's other works, I was struck by the time and attention that he had devoted to this series. His recording and interpretation seems almost obsessive. But once I left the museum and was making my meandering way back down the steep hill into downtown Zurich, my thoughts wandered from the portraits I had just seen to the time that Godé-Darel and Hodler had spent together. And I wondered what other purpose those sessions filled for them. How did they use that time? Did they talk about his future without her? Or did they spend it simply, in contemplation? I like to imagine Godé-Darel's gaze focused on a point somewhere off the canvas, and that somehow, freed of the need to look at each other and to talk of worldly things, that somehow their talk would have been transformed into something beautiful, making something unique of the last hours they spent together.

Alberto

But what about Alberto? Did he find his family? Were they reunited before he died? These are the questions that my medical students hound me with. Frustrated by my discussion of the importance of connections and the value of a life review, they urge me, with diminishing patience, to tell them how Alberto's story ends.

As we were working on locating Alberto's family, he gave us a clue to understanding his story, although none of us recognized it at the time. My Spanish vocabulary was hopelessly inadequate to tell him about his diagnosis, so we had relied on a professional translator to help us do this. But Alberto's reaction to her translation was bewildering. His demeanor as she spoke was almost casual, as if he didn't take her seriously. He seemed sad, but in a detached, almost distracted way. The most dire information—and there was plenty of it—was met with stolid acceptance, nods, and half-smiles. Alberto's nonchalance was particularly odd, given what I knew about this translator, who tended toward hyperbole and theatricality. Not knowing the script she was following, you might have thought that Alberto was hearing about the diagnosis of a distant cousin.

So we brought in another resident, Ricardo Gonzales, who spoke fluent Spanish. Alberto's response to Ricardo was no different, but at least Ricardo could give us a sense of what Alberto was thinking. Alberto, Ricardo said, had done some "very bad things" ("*hechos muy malos*") in his past, and his recent diagnosis was a sort of repayment for past sins. It was almost a relief, in a way, because Alberto had been expecting it, or something like it. It didn't matter that there's no scientific association between sins and glioblastoma, or that his exposure to pesticides as a farmworker was a more likely culprit. Alberto had an explanation, and buried in it was a clue that might have helped us to understand his past and find his family, if we had recognized it.

In the meantime, we were facing other difficulties. We had been trying to get in touch with Alberto's family as he had begged us to. When one of Alberto's drinking buddies visited the day Alberto was admitted, he was able to tell the night nurse that he thought Alberto had family living in Lancaster, Pennsylvania. It wasn't much of a lead, but we assigned one of our third-year medical students, Angela, to do some detective work. Still, after hours of sleuthing and a call to a friend of a friend who lived in Lancaster, we came up with nothing.

To make matters worse, it turned out that the Social Security number that Alberto had given to the social worker was incorrect. The verification process took a while, as it often did, and so it wasn't until the fourth day of Alberto's hospitalization that the social worker came into the doctors' conference room and slid into a chair, looking perplexed. The Social Security number Alberto gave was real, and it was assigned to someone of the same age, gender, and ethnicity as Alberto. But that person had a different name.

So was the Social Security number wrong? That would have been an unlikely coincidence. Or was Alberto really someone else?

By this point I think we were all more than a little disheartened. After all, Alberto had given us what should have been a simple request—to find his family. That was all that mattered to him. He didn't want to be cured, and he didn't expect us to prolong his life. He didn't even have ambitions to go home. He only wanted to see his family one more time. And we hadn't even managed that.

Finally, one of us (I can't remember who) put everything together. The name that matched the Social Security number wasn't

Alberto's, so "Alberto" must have been an alias. Then we went back to our search in Lancaster, this time using the name that matched Alberto's Social Security number. That surname was more common, but now we also had first names—of his entire family. And this time we found them, all of them, living in a large doublewide trailer outside of town.

In a burst of creativity, our social worker managed to find funds from the local migrant farmworkers union to fly Alberto's family to Iowa City and to put them up in a motel on Route 6, near the hospital. That reunion was worth all of the time and energy we had devoted. They arrived midmorning as we were rounding on our patients, and we had emerged from another patient's room to find them milling around at the nurses' station. His mother, two brothers, and sister, exactly as billed.

Alberto's family spent the better part of a week with him before he died, and over the course of that week his story emerged. He had come north from Guatemala about eight years before and found work in a computer assembly plant in St. Louis. He had applied for a green card and eventually became a citizen, receiving a Social Security card that carried the number that he had given us. Over the next few years he brought his family with him, including his mother, and they all got green cards.

All was well until Alberto was involved in some sort of trouble. His mother wasn't clear on the details. As she told the story through an interpreter, she kept looking at his twin brothers for confirmation at key points, but they looked away. I had the sense that they had been over this ground many times before. In any case, Alberto had gone to Canada for a while under an assumed name, and then, finally, came back as Alberto. He took odd jobs, traveling around the Midwest, working here and there, largely in menial labor jobs. Always, though, he would send money to his family in St. Louis and later to Lancaster when they moved there.

They were sad to see him when they did, of course, particularly since Alberto's diagnosis was a surprise to them. But they also realized how lucky they were to have had the chance to see him before he died. And certainly, Alberto's amazement at seeing his mother appear in his doorway was infectious. I think for all of us, this was a rare opportunity to feel like we had done something special, giving a patient a last chance to fulfill his wish and reconnect with family.

FOUR

Jerry

Asking Forgiveness and Making Amends

Jerry

I never actually took care of Jerry, and he didn't actually die. At least, not officially, in the hospital's record system. But Jerry did exist, and he did die. And in some database, somewhere, there was a mark next to his name that recorded his passing. Whoever made that mark didn't spend any time mourning his death, though. And the same, unfortunately, was probably true for almost everyone who had known him. Jerry wasn't a Mafia boss, a war criminal, or a child molester, but he might as well have been because we had concealed his official record in order to protect him.

For over ten years, Jerry had been one of the directors of the hospital's food service program, managing a large staff of cooks, servers, dieticians, and transport workers. In that time, Jerry had become widely known for a combination of laziness and boorish behavior that made him widely feared and universally hated. He would verbally abuse staff indiscriminately, making no allowances, even, for the elderly women who volunteered in the cafeteria. He would make capricious staffing decisions, assigning evening and weekend shifts seemingly at random. "Seemingly" because it became apparent, eventually, that these assignments were influenced by bribes and other favors. Jerry would give the easiest assignments to a small group of friends—all men—whom he had grown up with. The other assignments, and particularly weekends and holidays, would go to the rank and file, mostly to women.

And there were other stories, as if further evidence of his ruthlessness were needed, which were even less flattering. Once a bribe was handed over, Jerry would renege, increasing the asking price. Jerry would demand, and not infrequently receive, sex in exchange for jobs or favorable evaluations that could lead to a raise. He seemed to have worked hard to be worthy of his poor reputation.

Jerry also had a long history of alcohol abuse, drinking as much as a fifth of liquor every day for many years. He had a history of using other drugs, too, although that was in his distant past. How much of his behavior was the result of alcohol abuse was unclear. He was never drunk at work, as far as I heard. But perhaps in light of his numerous other transgressions, showing up at work inebriated simply didn't warrant comment.

Although the effect of his alcoholism on his work wasn't obvious, at least to me, its impact on his health could not have been more plain. The cumulative effects of his drinking had gradually scarred his liver, producing abnormal lab tests of his liver's function, then intractable gastritis, and finally ascites—large amounts of fluid in the abdomen surrounding the internal organs. The manifestations of that progressive destruction were traced in the stacks of medical records he had accumulated.

By the time he was forty-eight years old, Jerry had developed end-stage liver cirrhosis, which is an irrevocable death sentence, at least without a liver transplant. And because Jerry continued to drink, he effectively forfeited his place on the transplant list, instead pushing any remaining healthy liver tissue beyond its normally impressive capacity for regeneration. During the last several years before I met him, Jerry's cirrhosis had gained momentum like a boulder accelerating down a steep slope.

When he was hospitalized for the last time, he had reached the steepest part of that slope. Over the past several months, he had developed esophageal varices, which are abnormal veins in the esophagus that become engorged with blood that cannot pass through a thickened, scarred liver. Varices generally do not cause symptoms until they rupture. But when that happens, the result is appalling and catastrophic bleeding, typically with violent vomiting of bright red blood. It is often fatal.

In an attempt to reduce that risk, Jerry's gastroenterologist had initiated a course of sclerotherapy—injecting an irritant into the walls of the veins—that she hoped would cause them to become less fragile. Sclerotherapy has since fallen out of favor as a first-line treatment, and indeed those procedures proved to be only minimally effective in Jerry's case. But any treatment of varices is generally little more than a delaying tactic anyway.

Jerry would eventually have a major bleeding episode, we knew, which Jerry's gastroenterologist didn't think he could survive. His liver function was too weak, she said, to give his blood enough ability to form clots, and his overall health was too frail to withstand a major bleeding episode. So she thought that sometime in the next year he would have a massive bleed that would almost certainly be fatal.

But Jerry was lucky—some thought undeservedly so. In what proved to be an improbable stroke of good fortune, he began to experience the initial symptoms of a variceal bleed while he was at work at the hospital. He became lightheaded and fell to the floor in a hallway just outside the emergency room, where the resident made an early, and astute, diagnosis. Within thirty minutes of his first symptoms, the ER staff had used a large inflatable balloon to control the bleeding and an endotracheal tube connected to a ventilator to ensure that Jerry could continue to breathe.

He was transferred to the surgical intensive care unit, where he was given blood and platelets, and also plasma to temporarily restore his blood's ability to form clots. To everyone's surprise, Jerry's bleeding stopped, the balloon was removed, and his gastroenterologist was able to try a new technique—banding—to try to control his varices. His condition stabilized, he was transferred out of the ICU. Preparations were underway to discharge him as soon as we were sure that the bleeding had stopped.

But any celebration was cut short when Jerry developed hepatorenal syndrome, a complication of cirrhosis characterized by kidney failure that is both very difficult to reverse and universally fatal if it is not. The team caring for him was gravely concerned. They knew that the subtle decrease in kidney function apparent in a blood test could become full-blown renal failure and cardiac collapse very quickly. They would need to implement a plan to try to protect his kidney function as best they could, while fending off some of the other threats—bleeding, infection, delirium—that Jerry would face. As the team shifted from discharge planning to an intensive, and probably extended, plan of treatment, they realized that they had a new problem that they had never had to deal with before.

In the forty-eight hours since his discharge from the ICU, Jerry had been obstinately refusing to eat anything from his food tray. Convinced that the food service staff—his employees—had spit in his food, or worse, he was subsisting on crackers and small tubs of margarine stocked at the nurses' station. Jerry was not someone who harbored those sorts of fears quietly. He picked fights with the dietary staff who delivered his trays, occasionally accusing them of trying to poison him, but more often complaining about the meals. His tray was delivered late, he said, and removed too soon. And his food was cold, or tasteless, or too salty, or not salty enough.

To be fair, Jerry's fears were not without foundation. Most of the food service staff probably had grievances against him that would have justified at least some of the sabotage that Jerry imagined and probably some that he didn't. Indeed, there were rumors circulating that the food service staff had done many of the things that Jerry accused them of. But those were only rumors, as far as I could tell. My impression was that the staff who delivered trays were, if not sympathetic, then at least distantly courteous. But Jerry's fears grew unchecked until they filled the ward like a collective paranoid delusion.

In fact, Jerry's beliefs might actually have been a paranoid delusion caused by a syndrome called hepatic encephalopathy, which can produce disorientation, personality changes, and irrational beliefs. The possibility that his fears could have been a symptom seemed to have a two-sided effect on the way that we all responded to his complaints. On one hand, we seemed to be more skeptical about the truth of his claims, dismissing them more quickly—as a symptom—than we might otherwise have. On the other hand, though, a medical explanation made us more sympathetic to Jerry's fears. The result was that we responded to him, I think, much as one might respond to a child who is convinced that there are monsters under his bed—with a sort of dismissive sympathy.

That was not an attitude to which Jerry responded well, however. By the time I was called in as a consultant, after Jerry had been hospitalized for a week, the situation had deteriorated substantially. He hadn't been eating anything from the hospital's food trays, I learned, and had instead been placing orders to local restaurants that delivered to the hospital. And these meals had rapidly become a threat to his health, as their high salt content made his ascites worse and pushed his kidneys beyond their capacity. Even worse, Jerry had threatened to leave the hospital despite his doctors' advice that doing so would almost certainly be fatal. In fact, he probably would have left if he had had the strength, but after a week spent almost entirely in bed, he had become so deconditioned that even a walk across his room left him winded.

The layout of Jerry's ward was a series of branching corridors leading to identical alcoves that all fit together like a rabbit warren. And so when I went to see Jerry late on a Friday afternoon, I wasn't surprised that I couldn't find his room number. I circled the unit until, exasperated, I caught the attention of a harried nurse. Barely slowing down, she pointed into the alcove right in front of me at a room whose number, I realized, had been covered over with a rough DO NOT DISTURB sign, handwritten in chunky black letters.

"His wife put that sign up," she explained. "To keep people out and to hide the room number, which also keeps people out." She shrugged, smiled, and vanished into the adjacent room.

I knocked on the door as I opened it and went in—a standard busy-doctor-saving-time maneuver. A curtain was pulled around one of the beds, and the other seemed to be empty. I called Jerry's name, in a conversational tone at first and then more emphatically, thinking, somehow, that a more assertive approach would be best. When he didn't answer, I leaned around the coarse mesh curtain pulled around his bed. Jerry looked up, furious, shouting "Get the fuck out!" I realized that Jerry was using the bedpan, and the curtain was closed to prevent the sorts of incursions that I had just perpetrated. In just a few seconds, and with the best of intentions, I had become just another one of those people who were trying to make his life as miserable as possible.

I apologized as I retreated to the hallway, but it wasn't really a sincere apology. I was even a little amused. And I realized then that the stories I had been hearing about Jerry had left a residue of aversion in me as well. Not as thick, certainly, as for those who had worked with him. Still, I wondered whether I'd be able to give him the open-minded support that he needed.

So when I went back to Jerry's room ten minutes later, I was, perhaps, even more courteous than I would have been with another patient. Partly, I wanted to show him that he could trust me, that I really wasn't like the others. But I also wanted to prove to myself that I could put those stories aside, at least for a few minutes.

Seated on the empty bed across from Jerry, I understood immediately how he had been able to intimidate the fifty or so food service staff who worked for him. Despite a year of progressive illness and a decade or more of hard drinking, and worn down further by a grueling weeklong hospitalization, Jerry was still imposing. He was broad-beamed and easily six feet tall. His bare feet rested flat on the tile floor as he sat hunched over a rolling tray pulled up to the side of his bed. The way the late winter sunlight in an otherwise dark room caught his reddish-blond hair and hard face made him seem, I thought uncharitably, like a giant hunkered down in his cave.

Despite the unfavorable first impressions that we each had of one another, though, our conversation was surprisingly amicable. Jerry in particular was strangely conciliatory. He began by apologizing, as if he wanted to see whether I was someone he might be able to use, I thought. Someone, that is, who he needed to cultivate. Again, I realized, my preconceptions seemed impossible to set aside.

He hadn't been himself lately, he said. He'd been more irritable than usual, and he had a lot on his mind. It occurred to me then, as it had to others in the ICU, that this was a man whose daily routine had included a fifth of liquor and who was now stone-cold sober. Whatever pacifying effects alcohol had provided were now washed away.

I advanced this theory gently, almost as a peace offering, suggesting it as one possible explanation of his recent disagreements and troubles. As I did, though, Jerry ducked his head and squinted just a bit, like a fighter circling an opponent. I realized that whatever rapport I thought we had developed had disappeared in an incautious instant.

"Everyone always talks about my drinking. That it's too much, that I'm killing myself. That I'm killing my liver." His initial conversational tone had risen to near gale force. "And everyone's saying the same thing about a fifth a day. Where the hell did they get that? Some idiot medical student came up with that and you're all passing it around as gospel. How come no one ever asked me how much I was drinking? Huh?" He paused for a moment, not to calm down, as I had hoped, but just to get his breath.

One of the nurse's aides, Jeff, who had been a state high school wrestling finalist three years in a row, ducked around the curtain out of Jerry's view. Because of his size, Jeff had been assigned as the unofficial guard on Jerry's room. He raised an eyebrow—just checking, was I OK? I nodded, imperceptibly I thought, but perhaps not. Jerry swiveled to follow my gaze, but Jeff was gone. And when Jerry turned back to me, he seemed distracted, as if he couldn't quite figure out where he had left off.

So rather than pursue the issue of his drinking, I made a bid to establish my own usefulness. I told Jerry, maybe a bit grandly, that I had been asked to create an arrangement that would give him his privacy, or at least enough privacy to let him stay in the hospital. I was, I said, a sort of "fixer." And while that description was, perhaps, a bit ostentatious, it seemed to work for Jerry. At least it was a term he understood and one that he respected. So we got down to business and I offered my best solution, which was to give him an alias in the hospital medical record system. That would make him invisible to the food service staff, I said.

That is, until one of the staff came to deliver a tray and recognized him, Jerry pointed out. We pondered this problem for a silent moment, and then Jerry suggested the other half of the solution. We should put him in respiratory isolation, he said, which would require food service staff to leave his trays at the nurse's station. That ruse, we both recognized, would also limit entry by others from the housekeeping staff. So in a few minutes we had a solution that left Jerry visibly more relaxed. And I left his room that evening with an unaccustomed feeling of accomplishment. Jerry would stay in the hospital as long as he needed to, and he would do so by way of a mechanism that, I hoped, would make life easier for all of us.

In fact, the solution that Jerry and I had created proved to be remarkably successful. Jerry became more calm, and was even civil to the nursing staff. The nurses and others on the ward began to relax. And the atmosphere of the ward slowly began to return to normal. Jerry still perceived a threat, and continued to worry that his food was being adulterated, but at least he could hold those fears in check.

And as things returned to normal, Jerry's wife, Jess, began to visit more often, although she seemed to spend more time at the nurses' station than she did with Jerry. That's where I met her several days later. She was small, about half Jerry's size, but somehow more substantial. Solid and businesslike, she seemed to resemble the block letters on the sign outside Jerry's door. Knowing what I did about Jerry's history, my first impression was that this was a woman who probably could stand up to him. It was only after we had been talking for a few minutes that I registered that she was wearing the hospital's drab brown food service uniform. Not only had she endured Jerry as a husband, but also, apparently, as a boss.

The hospital was full and none of the nurses had a free moment, so their break room was empty. Jess and I ducked in and I closed the door behind us. I said I'd been surprised to see her, that I thought that Jerry was divorced. She shook her head, a little uncertainly. They were separated, actually. Jerry had been physically abusive, and although Jess hadn't pressed charges, she had moved out about two years ago. But they still saw each other at the hospital, of course. She hesitated. And, sometimes they saw each other socially. It was as if she wasn't sure how their relationship might be redefined now, and whether her attitude toward Jerry should be one of distance, rejection, tolerance, or forgiveness.

Our conversation turned then to Jerry's prognosis. I explained that this latest crisis was likely to be Jerry's last, and that the kidney failure that was keeping him in the hospital would likely be fatal. I thought he would die of kidney failure in the next several weeks, either here in the hospital or at home. Jess's reaction to my dismal prediction was a resigned sadness, uncomplicated by the shock or denial that often defines these sorts of conversations. She'd had the sense that things would eventually turn out this way, she said simply.

Jess was unsurprised, too, by Jerry's increasingly frequent requests to be discharged home. He'd begun to see through the tepid reassurances of his doctors and nurses, and I think he'd realized, finally, that he was going to die. He didn't want to die in the hospital or in a nursing home; he wanted to go home. But home, I knew, was little more than an empty house on the edge of town. Alone, with no one to help him and care for him, Jerry's last days at home would be wretched and grim.

Jess looked uncomfortable as I said this, and I asked whether she'd thought about whether she would take him in. And so we talked about what she should do. Or more precisely, we talked about what she was obligated to do (very little), and about what she could do (a great deal), and how to choose between the two.

This question must have been one that she had considered thoroughly because she had an answer ready. She would be willing to take him in, she said, if he offered several apologies. To her, and to a few of the staff with the most significant grievances. One man whose wife he had had an affair with. And a woman who, for reasons no one understood, bore the brunt of unfair work assignments. These apologies wouldn't have to be detailed and wouldn't even have to be heartfelt. But, Jess said, he would need to make the effort. It was as if the complicated economics of their relationship had been reduced to a single coin, this apology, which then became their sole medium of exchange.

Was it really that simple, I wondered? And was Jess really willing to take Jerry into her home in payment for even a token apology? That puzzled me. I couldn't see that such a simple gesture, a gesture that might well have been artifice, could have created a truce so neatly.

But I was more surprised by what she said next. I had asked her whether she was going to have this conversation with Jerry, and she said she already had. Dozens of times over the past week in the hospital. She couldn't have been more transparent, she said, about what she wanted from him. And Jerry, it seemed, couldn't have made it more plain that he wouldn't apologize. Ever.

Asking Forgiveness and Making Amends

There were many aspects of Jerry's history that were a mystery, but the most inscrutable, to me, was his refusal to apologize. I simply couldn't understand why Jerry wasn't willing to offer the apologies that Jess seemed to expect.

A few apologies would have been appropriate, I thought. And expedient. Indeed, if a few simple apologies could have helped him to leave the hospital, shouldn't that have been compellingly obvious to Jerry? He of all people should have understood the utility of an apology, even if that apology wasn't heartfelt. I was cynical enough to wonder, then, why he wouldn't even fake an apology. But he wouldn't.

His refusal to apologize puzzled me, too, because there is an almost ritualistic expectation of asking forgiveness near the end of life. Certainly, this is true of the last rites of the Catholic, Anglican, and Eastern Orthodox churches. Some form of confession and penance, the anointing of the sick (extreme unction) and the final Eucharist, or viaticum (provisions for the journey) form the foundation of absolution at the end of life. (It is a foundation, though, that some have eschewed. Pietro Perugino, for instance, was a Florentine master painter who taught Raphael, among others. Dying of plague, Perugino reportedly refused to send for a priest to administer the last rites, saying that he was curious to know what would happen to someone who dies without receiving the viaticum.)

Literature, too, reminds us of the value of efforts to atone for past misdeeds. There is, for instance, the poor unnamed woman in *Oliver Twist* whose last act is to try to atone for her theft, years before, of the locket that would have been the key to Oliver's parentage. And there are cinematic examples as well. In a wonderful French film, *Le Crabe-Tambour* (1977), a dying French naval captain tries to arrange a final rendezvous with a war hero who had been court-martialed unfairly, due in large part to the cowardice of the captain and others who refused to testify on his behalf.

Nowhere, though, are apologies so much a part of tradition—carefully scripted and choreographed—as they are in the last statements of inmates on death row. As I was writing this chapter, three Texas death-row inmates were executed within the space of a week or so. Robert James Anderson, convicted of the murder of a five-year-old girl: "To Audrey's grandmother, I am sorry for the pain I have caused you for the last 15 years and your family. I have regretted this for a long time. I am sorry." And Mauriceo M. Brown, convicted of a gang-related murder: "I am sorry you lost a brother, loved one, and friend." And Derrick O'Brien, convicted of rape and murder: "I am sorry. I have always been sorry. It is the worst mistake that I ever made in my whole life."

But the vividness of these examples is misleading, and suggests that such apologies occur only under exceptional circumstance, prompted by serious misdeeds. In fact, many of my patients—most of whom have led lives that that were generally unobjectionable—take a moment to apologize. What do my patients have to apologize for?

There are past misdeeds, certainly. I took care of an elderly man whose wife had long since died. There was a minor uproar one afternoon when he told his daughter that once, forty years before, he had been unfaithful to his wife (her mother). But there was less of a disturbance, oddly, a few days later when he apologized for what he said was another infidelity. The family seemed to have reached a tacit agreement to treat the second confession as the product of delirium.

Indeed, it's likely that none of us has apologized as fully as we might have. If that seems overreaching, consider for a moment the burdens that come with caring for someone with a serious illness near the end of life. For the family of someone with advanced cancer, for instance, there are physical burdens of caregiving. And families shoulder social burdens as well, including disrupted relationships and routines. There are psychological burdens of sadness and grief. And there are economic burdens associated with lost income, and the additional costs of the patient's health care, which even the best insurance never seems to cover entirely. All of these stresses can lead patients to believe they've become burdensome to friends and family.

When I was a resident, I took care of a patient in his sixties who had been left severely disabled by a stroke. He was disheartened not only by his physical weakness, but by the burden that his frailty placed on his wife, who was ten years his junior. Just as they were thinking about retirement, he said, this stroke had cost him his job and created a second, full-time caregiving job for his wife. No longer a husband, a partner, he had become work.

Without thinking, I mentioned a passage in a book I had just read, Harold Brodkey's *This Wild Darkness: The Story of My Death*. In it he apologized to his wife, Ellen, for being so much work. Ellen paused, Brodkey recalls, and then told him that he had always been a lot of work. The kind of work had changed, she said, but he had always been work. I paused for a moment, suddenly unsure whether I had said too much. But my patient rewarded my literary allusion with a sad, lopsided smile. Something in that anecdote, somehow, seemed to cheer him.

Motivations for an Apology

Why apologize? Of course, my patients' motives vary according to their circumstances. And they're too numerous, really, to fit into a taxonomy. But there are, I think, some overarching themes.

Some, I suppose, hope to make a form of restitution. But sometimes my patients aren't hoping to fix a mistake as much as they're hoping for a sense of closure. I took care of another patient, James, who had abandoned his wife and infant son many years before. He was vague about his reasons for leaving them. He wasn't ready to settle down, he said. At least, that was his packaged and well-worn summary of what was, I imagine, a much more complex and nuanced choice. Whatever his reasons, though, he had left. Disappeared. For a while, James told me, he would send money home. But as his shame subsided, those checks became increasingly infrequent, finally stopping altogether.

James and his wife eventually divorced. Or, rather, she divorced him, sending the legal papers to the return address of his last check. She soon remarried and so did he, years later. And at some point he got in touch with his son. They struck up a relationship of sorts. Distant, from the sound of it, but polite, their interaction seemed to be based mostly on an annual exchange of news around the holidays.

I took care of James briefly when he enrolled in our hospice program and found out about his history only indirectly, from our social worker. His past was distant history, we thought. His ex-wife had died a few years previously, and his son was grown, married, with children of his own.

Yet, our social worker noted, James had never apologized. Not to his ex-wife, nor to his son. She thought that he should. She didn't envision some sort of tearful reconciliation. I don't think she even imagined that an apology would have any effect at all on James's relationship with his son. All she wanted, she said, was for James to have the sense that he had closed that chapter of his life.

I wasn't so sure. I saw those events thirty or forty years ago as distant history, and something that James had almost forgotten. Moreover, I argued, what would be the point of an apology? It would, I thought, be superfluous at best. Worse, it might disrupt what I saw as a fragile alliance between father and son that I'd hoped might grow stronger over whatever time James had left.

I remember that we discussed this question in team meeting one Wednesday for fifteen or twenty minutes, an eternity for a busy hospice team. Still, we couldn't agree. It came down to a fundamental disagreement between the social worker's conviction that James needed a sense of closure, on one hand, and my fear of opening old wounds, on the other.

It was actually our volunteer coordinator who suggested that perhaps we should just ask our patient what he wanted. We could even describe the potential benefits of an apology, as we saw them, as well as the potential harms. And that, finally, was what we decided to do.

James's nurse was the next to make a home visit, and when she asked him, he agreed immediately. Interestingly, she used the language that the social worker had suggested, but he was careful to correct her. It wasn't, he said, that he wanted to close that chapter of his life. The mistake that he made would always be with him. And he couldn't look at a Christmas card from his son without thinking, one more time, about how he had acted. So he wasn't "closing" anything.

Instead, he told her, he felt he needed to apologize in order to tie everything together. He used the analogy of a jumble of objects that are difficult to carry. He saw a formal apology as a way of tying those objects together in a package. He'd continue to "carry" that package with him. But the apology made it more neat somehow, and more contained.

In the end, the apology that we had debated so hotly turned out to be little more than a note on a small greeting card. His nurse was there, in fact, when James wrote it. The two of them talked a little about what the note should say, so she had a sense of what was in it. It was short, she said. No more than a sentence or two. It said, simply, that James was sorry for all the hurt he had caused.

Was our social worker right? I think she was. She thought, and the nurse agreed, that James seemed more peaceful, less distracted, after he put that note in the mail. So for him, an apology wasn't about revisiting the past, and it wasn't about asking for forgiveness, as I had imagined. And it certainly wasn't about making amends. It was, as he'd said, more a way of tying up loose ends.

For other patients, a desire to apologize seems to be driven by religious convictions. I took care of an elderly African-American woman once, a leader in her church and her community. Dying of advanced breast cancer, Gloria was in our hospice program and had, perhaps, a month at most to live. In that time, she told us, she wanted to make sure that she was "right" with God. And that meant, for her, being "right" with everyone she knew. So when Gloria had visitors, and when she spoke on the phone with friends and family members, she would make a point of asking whether there was anything outstanding between them.

Our nurse and our social worker heard or saw several of these conversations, and said they followed more or less the same format. Gloria would say that she didn't have much time left. Weeks or months, maybe. She would wait for the other person's protestations to subside, and then she would say she wanted to meet Jesus as clean and as pure as she came into this world. So Gloria wanted to know whether there was anything between them, whether there were things she had done or said that she needed to be clear of, and to get that stain of sin off of her.

I never witnessed one of these conversations, but our nurse and social worker both had roughly the same impression. It was a beautiful moment to watch, and to be a part of, they said. But it was also, they admitted, a bit of a farce. There was no real opportunity to apologize, they thought. And I understood what they meant. Gloria's friends and family would have to have been churlish indeed to tell a dying woman—particularly one as blame-free as Gloria seemed to be—that she owed them an apology.

But I think we all missed the point. Gloria knew, I'm sure, that her visitors and callers wouldn't ask for an apology. I'm also sure that if she had ever owed an apology to anyone, she had offered it long ago. No, the real script underlying these stylized exchanges was simply the offer and its rejection, an almost liturgical call and response whose rhythm signified an obligation discharged. It was not at all the farcical offer of an apology that we'd seen at first, but rather a more quiet, solid reassurance for everyone that any transgression had been forgiven.

If Gloria's apology was a way of documenting forgiveness, for other patients an apology offers a way to shape or control how they will be remembered. Sam was not terminally ill by most definitions. Although he had several serious illnesses—diabetes, heart disease, mild kidney failure—that would probably limit his life expectancy, none of them by itself was likely to be fatal. Yet he behaved as if he were as close to death as most of my patients are.

About three years before I met him, Sam had suffered a cardiac arrest. His heart stopped and he was (almost) dead. But he happened to be at the right place at the right time—in the clinic of a major medical center's outpatient surgery department—where all of the staff and equipment necessary to resuscitate him were, literally, in the next room. So he survived that episode and had a defibrillator implanted that would shock his heart back into a normal rhythm if necessary.

I knew most of that history from one of the fellows who had seen Sam in the geriatrics clinic on previous visits. And so one day in clinic, when we had a little extra time because we were waiting for his daughter to park the car, I asked him about the time that he almost died. In particular, I was curious about whether that experience had changed him. Not many of us get a second chance, I said. Had he done anything different the second time around?

He laughed self-consciously. At first, he told us, he had made all manner of promises, a few of which he had managed to keep. He stopped smoking, for instance, and he lost about fifty pounds. But other promises that demanded more far-ranging changes proved too easy to forget. He told himself, for instance, that he would start going to church regularly, that he would be more active as a leader in his community, and that he would volunteer for a local civic organization. He managed to do a few of these things but six months later he had fallen back into his old habits.

That's not entirely true, though, Sam admitted. There was one change that had stuck. It wasn't a large one and, indeed, it wasn't even the result of a resolution that he had been conscious of making. He realized, though, that after his "accident" he was much more careful—almost superstitiously so—about walking away from arguments or disagreements. He had become vividly aware, he said, that any argument could, if he were to die suddenly, define the way that people would remember him. He would be remembered not by his previous sixty-plus years, but by the last thing that he'd said or done. So after he was discharged from the hospital with his defibrillator, he would take care to "batten down the hatches" of any argument before going to sleep at night.

This process always, or almost always, involved an apology. Sometimes it was a direct apology. More often, though, it was a conditional apology. "I'm sorry if what I said made it sound like . . ." or "I'm sorry if you thought I was implying that . . ." Sam's rule applied to arguments at home with his family, but even more often, he said, to disagreements at work. In fact, he had developed a reputation among coworkers for leaving late-night messages on their voicemail.

It surprised him, he said, how that small habit had transformed other people's opinions of him. Many people had said in general terms that he seemed "nicer," and "a better person" since his near-death. More than a few seemed to interpret that change in their own ways. They said that he seemed more at peace, that he had less of an ego, or—his favorite—that he had become more of a "people person," whatever that meant.

Sam told me this not because he believed any of it. On the contrary, he was quick to deny that his brush with death three years previously had made him better, wiser, or any different at all, except for this minor habit of never leaving things undone. He was more amused that such a little habit could be interpreted in such varied ways, and that it could be interpreted as such a dramatic change.

I stopped seeing patients in the geriatrics clinic a short time after that conversation, and I never spoke with Sam again. About two years later, though, I heard that he had been admitted to the ICU with a massive stroke. I went to see him but found him on a mechanical ventilator, heavily sedated and unaware of his surroundings. I heard, several days later, that he had died without waking up.

For any other patient I might have regretted those last days spent under a blanket of sedation, unable to interact with friends and family. But in his case, I'm reasonably sure that even if there were things left undone and unsaid, Sam's apologies, at least, were up to date.

Barriers to an Apology

All of these examples underscore the value of an apology. And they also illustrate apologies that seem natural, graceful, and easy. In that regard they're inspiring but not, I think, entirely representative.

I can think of several of my patients, for instance, who found apologies much more difficult. And these are the stories that I turn over in my mind as I think about Jerry's steadfast refusal to apologize to his wife and others. Is there, perhaps, something buried in these stories that might explain Jerry's odd reluctance?

For instance, I took care of a young woman once—Lisa—who was in her thirties. We learned, from hints in conversations with her, that she'd had a falling-out with her sister a year or so earlier. The two had been close, according to one of Lisa's friends, but were now estranged for reasons no one could explain. When I met her, Lisa was dying of breast cancer, a diagnosis that was extraordinary in someone so young. Her situation was so unusual, in fact, that we wondered if she had a genetic predisposition that her sister might share. And so we paid more attention to her relationship with her sister than we might have otherwise.

Lisa had been admitted to the oncology service with shortness of breath that proved to be caused by an infiltration of cancer around her heart. This condition—a malignant pericardial effusion—usually appears in the later stages of cancer and is almost always fatal. As it became clear that Lisa had no more than a week to live, we began to suggest that her widely scattered family should come if they could. But her father had died two years before and her mother, it turned out, was too ill to travel. That left Lisa's sister, who was teaching English in China. One morning Lisa's nurse told me that she and Lisa had spent the better part of the evening before on the phone with the hospital operator trying to get in touch with Lisa's sister. Apparently, she was teaching in a rural part of China where neither Internet access nor cell-phone service were readily available.

The two of them had not been successful that night, and by the time I went to see Lisa the next morning, she was frustrated, and frightened, too, that she would never be able to reach her sister. She was distraught enough, in fact, that she let slip a small bit of information about the events that had separated them. I could tell only that it was something minor at first, related to a disagreement about planning their father's funeral. But their disagreement grew over the course of a few months, fueled by poor communication, busy schedules, and, finally, by her sister's extended trip to China that separated them completely.

And now, it seemed, Lisa had waited too long. The hospital operator the night before had made some progress in locating the office of the organization that her sister worked for. But the operators' shifts had changed at 8 A.M., and the hospital switchboard had become much more busy. This, plus the time difference, meant that any further attempts would have to wait until the next evening.

Lisa became increasingly short of breath that day, and by evening the decision had been made to keep her comfortable. Her declining heart function and the effects of the medications we were giving her to ease her breathing had made her increasingly somnolent. She wasn't asleep but floated in a sort of half-waking state that seemed like a quiet delirium. In the end, a phone call proved to be impossible.

As it turned out, though, Lisa was able to offer an apology of sorts. I wasn't there that night but heard from her nurse that shortly past midnight, and not long before Lisa died, she became confused enough that she seemed to mistake one of the nurse's aides for her sister. She startled the aide by telling her that she was sorry, her nurse said. And, after some prompting from the nurse, the aide said that she was sorry, too.

If the barriers that Lisa faced seem daunting—and they were—at least her apology had a goal, a person to whom an apology was owed. Like Jerry's, her apology was, or should have been, relatively easy. It was an opportunity missed, irrevocably, through delay and avoidance. But sometimes an apology is simply not possible.

Rob was a Vietnam veteran I took care of once whose quiet, gentle manner was disrupted unpredictably by flashes of anger that would startle his family and frighten the nursing staff. He never talked to me about his time in Vietnam, at least not directly. But he did tell me once about a trip he had taken there a few years earlier. Rob worked as a landscaper and the winter was, for him, an extended furlough. So one winter he and two buddies from his Army days went to Vietnam for two months. They traveled, visiting the sites of firefights and casualties. And they also helped build a school and dig wells for several villages in an area where they had been stationed.

I tried to find out what motivated that trip and it turned out that it wasn't the first time Rob had been back to Vietnam. In fact, he had made a half-dozen or so trips over the past twenty years. Sometimes he'd go with a small group, and once he went alone. He went for varying periods of time, anywhere from two weeks to two months. Always, though, Rob said he'd try to do something "useful." For instance, he often spent his time building or working on other projects that made use of his skills.

We talked at length about what he did while he was there but very little, in contrast, about why he went. Rob would say, cryptically, only that he "owed" something to one village. Or that he "needed to do something" in another.

I never pressed him to tell me about what he felt he owed, or why. Those flashes of anger weren't far from my mind as we talked. I had been their focus on one occasion and had been surprised when Rob's gentle demeanor had disappeared, replaced by a snarling expression and parade-ground voice. That outburst subsided as quickly and as inexplicably as it had begun, followed by a contrite apology. But it had left me and, I suspect, others, with a reluctance to intrude. Still, I've always assumed, based on stories that other patients have told me, that whatever happened in those rice fields and villages was something Rob felt he needed to atone for.

The barrier that Rob faced was even greater, in a way, than the one that separated Lisa and her sister. The people to whom Rob felt he owed an apology were quite possibly dead, as were their families. And of course they were anonymous. Faces perhaps dimly remembered, and entirely unreachable in any case. And replaced instead in his memory by placeholders of obligation—village names, landmarks, and survey coordinates—to which he felt he owed something.

Faced with the challenge of making amends to people who were anonymous, Rob had developed a compromise, I think. He would go back to the same areas, to the same villages and valleys. And without knowing it, he'd meet the family members of those he had fought, or perhaps their children, or perhaps even the ex–Viet Cong themselves. But rather than apologizing directly, he would build schools. He would dig wells and he would teach children to speak English. Rob had, I thought, invented his own form of restitution.

And apparently he maintained records of that restitution that were as meticulous as his landscaping accounts had been. Although I never saw it, his wife told me later that Rob kept a scrapbook of pictures that he or others had taken, pictures of the school he had helped to build or of people drawing water from the well he helped to dig. Pictures of the children he taught. I like to think that this scrapbook was a sort of balance sheet that summarized his progress toward whatever redemption he thought he could achieve.

Atonement Through Suffering and Death

Do these stories provide an explanation for Jerry's reluctance to offer an apology? I don't think they do. If anything, they reinforce my sense that Jerry missed an obvious opportunity that many of my other patients, like Lisa or Rob, would have been overjoyed to have been offered.

This is one of the aspects of Jerry's story that I find so frustrating. Many of my patients manage to overcome vast barriers to apologize to others. And yet for Jerry the opportunity could not have been easier. His transgressions were certainly obvious, and they were numerous. The people he had injured were all around him and were, moreover, willing to accept an apology. Why, then, was Jerry so reluctant to apologize?

In fact, I had already stumbled across one possible answer, but I hadn't recognized it at the time. When I first met Jess, in that conversation in the nurses' break room, I had asked her whether she thought that Jerry would ever apologize. She said she didn't think he would. He didn't see why he should have to apologize to anyone. He wasn't even fifty years old and he was dying, he'd told her. And not just dying peacefully, but suffering the indignities of a death due to cirrhosis, with an enormous belly like some circus freak. Wasn't he suffering enough? He was already being punished, why should he have to apologize, too?

As I thought back to that conversation with Jess, I wondered whether, perhaps, Jerry was refusing to apologize at least in part because he was already being punished for the things he had done. Was it possible that Jerry had connected his past behavior and his illness? Perhaps, I thought, he viewed his illness and its indignities, and his premature death, as adequate payment for whatever he had done.

At first it seemed farfetched to imagine that Jerry might construe his suffering and eventual death as a punishment for past transgressions and atonement for those transgressions. But I don't think that this view is so unusual.

When I was a resident, I took care of a young woman who had a rare form of cancer that arises in the back of the throat, invading the adjacent areas of the neck and sinuses. It's a very aggressive cancer and difficult to treat. It's also intensely debilitating because as it advances it interferes with the ability to swallow and to talk, and can cause severe pain.

I met Marta when she was admitted to our service for treatment of a sinus infection that was a result, probably, of a blockage caused by the tumor. The cancer itself had just been diagnosed a few weeks earlier, and she hadn't yet begun to receive treatment. So all of this was new to her. Marta was still trying to make sense of the diagnosis, asking, as many of my patients seem to, why this particular disease chose her.

When I first meet patients, time permitting, I usually ask what they know about their illness—what it is, how it affects them, and whether it's treatable or not. I also try to find out what they understand about its cause. That information in particular can help me sometimes to see what anthropologist Arthur Kleinman described as a patient's "explanatory model." Not only what their illness is, how it behaves, and its likely prognosis, but also where it came from.

And so on the night Marta was admitted, she told me she thought that her cancer had something to do with her "wild living" of ten to fifteen years ago. I didn't know what that wild living was, and I didn't ask her that night, partly because I was busy with other patients to see. But mostly I didn't want to ask questions that might legitimize her belief that she was somehow responsible for her cancer. And so I said simply, and with as much assurance as I could muster, that most of the time cancer was a matter of luck. Just as a tornado might rage through a town, destroying one house but leaving another untouched, I said, cancers like hers seemed to pick their victims at random.

I had intended my answer to be reassuring. Trying to sound confident and authoritative, I wanted to erase as completely as I could any notion that she was responsible for her illness. But Marta didn't seem to be listening. More specifically, she didn't seem to want to hear what I was saying. She wouldn't meet my gaze and instead looked down and to the side as if in embarrassment. I had the impression that I had just broken some unwritten cultural convention for which an acknowledgment was too embarrassing. Regardless, it was obvious that my explanation had done little to convince her that her cancer was not her fault.

My explanation wasn't a success, it turned out, because Marta had already become convinced that she was at least partly to blame. That was her understanding of her cancer's etiology in her explanatory model. That model had been reinforced, unfortunately, earlier that evening when she asked a well-meaning but bumbling medical student whether there might be any connection between her past behavior and her cancer. He explained that, in fact, there were certain viruses that increased the likelihood of certain kinds of cancer, including hers. So it was possible, he said helpfully, that she might have acquired such an infection years ago that would have put her at increased risk.

The next morning when the medical student related this conversation, the attending physician and I berated him for "blaming" Marta for her cancer. We believed that endorsing her belief was factually incorrect, and ethically wrong as well. We were also worried that the belief—however misguided—that she was in part to blame for the illness that would end her life would unnecessarily add to Marta's suffering.

So we marched grimly to her room on rounds the next morning, trailed by the now-sheepish medical student, expecting a long discussion to undo whatever harm he had caused. The attending physician recapitulated what the medical student had said, point by point. He acknowledged that the medical student's facts were correct, and that there are some cancers that arise because of a viral infection. But Marta's was not one of these, he told her. Hers was simple bad luck. With this, the attending concluded with exactly the sort of confident flourish that I had been trying to achieve the night before.

His delivery was certainly more impressive than mine had been, but it was not any more effective. Marta responded in much the same way as she had the night before, in fact. Looking down at her hands twined in her lap, she wasn't so much listening as she was waiting until the attending had finished his speech so she could say her piece.

And finally she did. After thinking and "praying on it" (she was deeply religious, a Baptist fundamentalist), she said she was sure, now, that her previous sins were in large part responsible for her cancer. It seemed that she didn't understand everything that the medical student told her, which was probably just as well. But she knew in her heart, she said, that some of her sins in the past had planted the seeds of her cancer. She said that she was grateful that God had spared her as long as He did. He didn't have to, she pointed out. Look at Herod or the Egyptians, struck down in their tracks. She had raised two wonderful daughters, and had a lot to be grateful for. But now it was time to pay for her past sins.

She said all this simply and calmly, as if she were describing a credit card bill for some wanton purchases that had come due. Her face was so placid, in fact, that at first I didn't truly register what she was saying. And when I did, finally, I was at a loss for how to respond.

At that moment, I think that all of the doctors on the team, and particularly the medical student, wanted to deny categorically that her past life played any role in producing the cancer that would end her life. On the other hand, she seemed to be finding an odd sort of comfort in the idea that she had caused her cancer, at least to some degree. I didn't understand how that could be. I thought that, if anything, her illness would have been made that much more difficult to bear by the belief that she was somehow responsible. But it was obvious that she found a profound peace in the idea that her cancer was a way for her to redeem herself and to erase the things she had done in the past.

The chaplain on our palliative care service, Lucy Pierre, often tells me that our patients see their illnesses as some form of punishment. Her response, she says, is to support their belief. Whatever they've done in the past, they've been redeemed by their illness. She can say this, somehow, with considerable authority. Only five feet tall, she is soft-spoken most of the time but can harness a voice of authority when it's needed.

It's more difficult for me to find a response, because that worldview is so different from mine. Still, we can usually arrive at some sort of compromise. That is, I can live with an explanatory model in which my patients place some of the blame for an illness on their past behavior, as long as it seems to serve a purpose for them, especially if they find it comforting, and if it helps them to make sense of the chaotic chance of whatever illness is going to end their lives. Even if I don't share beliefs like Marta's, I find I can treat them as one would treat another's cultural beliefs, not with full understanding or even agreement, but at least with respect.

When I hear stories like Marta's, I think that these patients are crafting narratives that complete their lives, narratives that make sense. There is blame and punishment, certainly. But there is also good fortune, for a time, the postponement of death. In fact, although these stories are, on the surface at least, about blame and punishment, it's noteworthy that many of my patients are grateful. They are not angry at dying young, but grateful for having been spared for so long. And so there is a sort of enveloping comfort even in narratives that center on a death as atonement for past wrongs.

But it is more difficult to accept these narratives, I find, when notions of blame and responsibility are tied to patients' suffering. This is where I find it impossible to sit back with the coolness of an ethnographic observer. As Marta's cancer progressed, she developed pain that proved to be impossible to manage. Despite escalating doses of morphine, the hospice nurse would find her in her apartment, curled on her threadbare sofa, unwilling to move and afraid to be moved.

The pain itself wasn't difficult to treat. The problem was that she would wait until the pain became unbearable and then take a very small dose of pain medication, much smaller than she needed. And then she would feel guilty, as if she had failed to atone because she had taken medication.

I realized that there was nothing we would be able to do that could erase her belief that her pain was somehow purifying and cleansing. Instead, we asked the hospice chaplain to talk with her, and he brought in a minister who had met her during her infrequent appearances at his church.

Together, they were able to convince her that the road to redemption was through prayer, not pain. They used an analogy that I've since used with several patients. They told her that her pain was a distraction from what was really important—prayer and salvation. She was letting herself be distracted, chasing after salvation on her own terms. She agreed with their message, eventually, and died about a month later, more comfortable—both physically and spiritually—than she had been for a very long time.

Jerry

After I met Jess, I became convinced that Jerry's refusal to apologize was somehow linked to a belief that he was already atoning through his suffering. I even wondered whether perhaps some of his fears of what the dietary staff might have been doing to his meals might be his way of amplifying that suffering. Perhaps he had convinced himself that the staff were already exacting their revenge and that, therefore, he was already paying for whatever wrongs he had done to them.

I had the chance to talk to Jess again late one afternoon about a week after Jerry had been transferred out of the ICU. By that time, his condition had deteriorated markedly. No longer alert, he had developed hepatic encephalopathy, as we had feared he would. He was only occasionally able to recognize Jess, and was frequently confused and combative, requiring near-constant supervision.

Against this backdrop, my second conversation with Jess had an oddly funereal feel. It was as if, I thought, we were discussing the content of a memorial service. I was trying to understand what drove Jerry to behave the way he did, but I was doing so more as a matter of closure and finality. And with a pathologist's sad certainty that it was too late to alter the course of events.

That afternoon, Jess told me more about Jerry's history that I hadn't known. For instance, Jerry grew up in a rural town, which was virtually owned by a small religious community that held exceptionally strict beliefs about sin and damnation. His father had served as the equivalent of a deacon—a sort of lay pastor—in their church, and so Jerry had been held to even higher moral standards than his friends had been.

His father had been abusive, she said. Not strictly speaking, she clarified, but by Jerry's account at least, he'd been a harsh disciplinarian. And Jerry got into trouble often. More often, it seemed, as he got older, until finally when he was about seventeen he ran away from home, lied about his age, and enlisted in the Army. He seemed to do well, reenlisting once, and then leaving at the end of his second tour. After a series of temporary jobs, he began working in the hospital food service, gradually working his way up the ranks.

So was Jerry religious, I asked?

No, Jess said. He hadn't been, at least as long as she'd known him. He didn't pray and didn't go to any church. But he never criticized her whenever she went to a church in their neighborhood. It was a different denomination than the one he'd been brought up in. Still, Jerry seemed to have some lingering respect for religion, or at least a wary deference. Her infrequent announcements that she was going to church had usually been greeted with, if not support, then a tacit acknowledgment that she, at least, was doing the right thing.

When I finally asked her, Jess said she thought that Jerry really did believe that his death was payment for past misdeeds. She was sure of it, in fact. It fit with the way he had been brought up, but more generally, it seemed to fit the way that he had lived his life. As if he were getting away with something, she said. As if he knew that, at some point, his luck would turn.

Jess seemed oddly pleased by this notion, or at least comforted by it. And so I asked her how it made her feel. Was Jerry's idea of atonement a substitute for the apology that she had asked for?

No, she admitted, it really wasn't. But then, nothing about their life together was exactly what she had asked for, she said wryly. They had had some good times together, for sure. Jerry could be gallant and stubbornly protective of her, for instance. But even those good times were slightly off-center, as if something weren't quite right. So she was used to making the best of what she had. And she would do that again now.

Jerry died a few days later. Although I suspect that Jess might eventually have been willing to care for him at home, there was no time to arrange for his discharge, and so he died in the hospital. But the memorial service was much larger than anyone expected, I heard. Perhaps people came out of respect for Jess, or out of a simple curiosity to see who else would take the time to come. Or perhaps Jerry's version of atonement had worked after all.

FIVE

Marie

Revenge and Forgiveness

Marie

I'd like to believe that the nearness of death imposes a truce that subdues—for a short time at least—all the feelings of anger and resentment that we live with every day. It seems that there ought to be something about the proximity of death that will help us to "forgive and forget," and that will produce a more genial, forgiving nature. Indeed, popular wisdom tells us that our awareness of impending death should induce us to become somehow better—more forgiving, more accepting—and less susceptible to the insults and slights that would have induced fits of fury only a few months before.

And that seems like a good thing. It would be a waste, wouldn't it, to spend one's last few days, or hours, rehearsing old insults and injustices? I'd like to believe that we'll all be able to depend on this transformation, and the freedom that it brings. And in fact many of my patients do manage a sort of unilateral disarmament, giving up bitterness and rancor and enjoying in exchange a sort of armistice with those around them. But that transformation isn't always effortless, and goodwill and forgiveness are not granted automatically.

Marie was a young woman whose relationship with her family was wild, unpredictable, and ultimately mystifying to most of us who knew them. For instance, when she went for a surgical procedure a few months before I met her, she had put her surgeon in an awkward position by forbidding him to discuss her care with her mother—an aggressive, domineering force of nature—or anyone else in her family. And on at least one occasion, her mother's visit degenerated into a loud disagreement that prompted the nurses on the floor to call hospital security to restore order.

Marie had a particularly aggressive form of polyarteritis nodosa (PAN), an autoimmune disease that has protean manifestations ranging from a rash and arthritis in many patients to kidney failure in an unfortunate few. At least in part because of the immunosuppressive drugs they must take, some patients with PAN also develop life-threatening infections. And in Marie's case, these drugs were what led to her current admission.

She had initially come to see her rheumatologist complaining of pain that seemed to be neuropathic—caused by nerve irritation—running down the backs of her legs. Although there are many potential causes of neuropathic pain, Marie also had weakness in her left leg, which is often the sign of a more serious problem. So her rheumatologist sent her for an emergency MRI, which revealed an extensive infection in her lower spine, with erosion of several vertebral bones, leaving her spine unstable and her spinal cord vulnerable. She was admitted for bed rest, antibiotics, and surgery to stabilize her spine.

Her rheumatologist knew all too well about Marie's difficult relationship with her family. Marie had been hospitalized three times in the past six months, and her family's fights, I later learned, had become legendary on the seventh floor, where she was usually admitted. So Marie's family situation was neither new nor surprising. It had become simply one of many chronic issues in Marie's care, like her immune status or her blood counts, which her physicians needed to work around carefully.

But during this hospitalization her rheumatologist had begun to sense that Marie's family situation was going to become an acute problem. Just as a chronic concern like a patient's low white blood count may become a crisis in the presence of an infection, Marie's family situation—a chronic concern—would become an acute problem if she were to lose the ability to make decisions for herself. If that happened, her rheumatologist realized, he would be forced to rely on Marie's family to make decisions for her. This was clearly something that Marie wouldn't want.

At the time, I was doing a fellowship in medical ethics at the University of Chicago, and I worked part-time as an ethics consultant at a small community hospital on the north side of the city. As part of my work there, I reviewed ethics cases with the residents and medical students from Northwestern University and provided consultative advice to the other physicians at the hospital. And so Marie's rheumatologist asked me to help determine who should make decisions about her care when she lost the ability to make decisions herself.

Unfortunately, I didn't get any of Marie's history from him. The only information I received came during a rather unhelpful phone call from his secretary, a brutally efficient woman who spoke in impatient monosyllables. So when I arrived on Marie's floor, I went looking for her medical chart. As it turns out, though, I only needed to ask Sheila, Marie's nurse, whom I had met the week before on another consult.

When I asked her why she thought the rheumatologist might have consulted me, Sheila just giggled. "He probably wants you to get rid of Marie's mother." She nudged me with her shoulder. "Quietly, you know? You can do that, right?" In retrospect, I think that Sheila had intuited exactly what Marie's rheumatologist wanted. Since that wasn't possible, though, Sheila told me instead what she knew about Marie's story.

Marie was thirty-four, she said, and had a master's degree in social work. She had worked, until very recently, as a medical social worker at another North Side hospital. She came from a large Baptist family, all of whom, it seemed, lived within a few square blocks nearby, just west of Wrigley Field. In addition to her parents, the family included two brothers and two—no, three—sisters, and an indefinite number of aunts, uncles, and cousins.

I don't know that theirs was ever a peaceful family. But Sheila said that it had become much more unruly when, just before graduating from social-work school, Marie announced to her family that she was gay. And that she was moving out of her grandmother's house, where she had been staying through school, and moving in with Rosalie, a divorced Puerto Rican woman, several years older, who was in her graduating social work class.

That was some ten years ago, and five years before her diagnosis of PAN. Since then, Marie and Rosalie had engaged in a sort of cold-war diplomacy with Marie's family. Rosalie would talk Marie into attending some family gathering, at which they would both feel noticeably unwelcome. There would be covert mutterings by a cousin followed by periods of uncomfortable silence, and occasional loud insults from Marie's father. And so they'd leave, vowing never to try again. But a month or two later Rosalie would try again, wanting still to be part of their family.

That awkward equilibrium was disrupted, first, by Marie's diagnosis, which led to skirmishes between Rosalie and Marie's mother over caregiving roles. Still, they managed to avoid a complete break until Rosalie was diagnosed with metastatic ovarian cancer. Her treatment options were limited, and the most aggressive of them involved extensive surgery that Rosalie refused. Over the next eight or nine months—time that was measured out by two or three of Marie's hospitalizations—Rosalie lost half her weight, becoming wasted and gaunt. She died less than a year after her diagnosis, in the hospice unit nearby at Northwestern.

These events proved—perhaps understandably—impossible for Marie's family to dismiss as coincidence. Two openly gay women were living in sin, as they saw it, and were both struck down by disease. This was clearly the will of God. And just as clearly, Marie's road to health lay in salvation. Marie's mother in particular wasn't shy about sharing this view with anyone who would listen.

This was not what Marie needed to hear, of course, and any semblance of family closeness evaporated for some time afterward. The next time Marie was hospitalized, her mother and a cousin came to visit, bringing the usual prayers for her salvation. That's when a fight erupted, and Marie threw a pitcher of water at the cousin. Sheila and another nurse intervened, called security, and had Marie's family removed.

At some point in Sheila's narrative, as I perched on the nurses'-station counter listening, I had noticed over Sheila's shoulder an angular woman leave Marie's room—her mother, presumably. She was severe-looking, in her sixties, with a hatchet nose and cheekbones like mallets, her shoulder-length grey hair tied back. She was wearing a thin black overcoat reaching almost to her feet. So as Sheila continued her story, it was this prejudiced and probably unfairly mean image that came to my mind whenever Sheila mentioned Marie's mother.

As I walked down the long hallway to Marie's room at the far end, that's the image that I conjured of Marie as well, a younger version of her mother. Less of a caricature, perhaps, but equally unprepossessing.

When I first met her, Marie was curled up at the head of her bed, using two hospital pillows as a backrest, arms wrapped around her legs and hands tucked back under her knees. She seemed smaller than she was, and certainly smaller than she would seem later, as I overheard an argument she would have a few days later with her mother over the phone, during which she'd seem to grow taller, wider, louder. Now, wrapped in a form-fitting black warm-up suit and a thin afghan shawl, with an orange silk scarf tying back spiky black hair, she seemed diminutive, contained, and more of a potential presence.

She had just emerged from a corrosive session with her mother, which she would tell me about several days later. Her posture, I came to understand later, was one of retrenching and regeneration. But I didn't see that at the time. From the doorway, I saw her coiled into a reclusive Q at one end of the bed, but I didn't see her hurt and loneliness. She looked to me like nothing so much as a swimmer about to unfurl, soar and plunge.

What misled me into seeing her as more vigorous than she was, I think, were her intense green eyes, eager and vehement at the same time. They seemed to contain all of the life and energy that weren't apparent in her bearing. Her eyes seemed to me to be those of someone both older and younger. An impish grandmother, say, or a precociously wise child.

I introduced myself and explained that her rheumatologist had asked me to help her decide who she'd want to make decisions for her. I also told her—briefly—what I'd learned from Sheila. Although I didn't realize it at the time, I think that I tuned my own demeanor to what I saw in her eyes—the energetic person she had been and would be again—rather than to the reclusive attitude that her body language suggested. And so as I introduced myself, I was more animated than I would normally have been, incongruously, if not inappropriately, so.

But it was this buoyancy that proved to be exactly what Marie needed. As we talked, and as I asked her questions to fill in some of the details that were missing from Sheila's account, Marie unfolded in stages. First cross-legged with elbows resting on knees and hands clasped and then, finally, sitting on the edge of the bed facing me, chin in hands. And that's the pose that I remember best—the one that she would assume whenever I came to visit her over the next few weeks.

The substance of that first conversation wasn't particularly complicated. We quickly decided that Marie should designate one of her friends to make health care decisions for her. In fact, we could probably have arrived at that conclusion in the first fifteen minutes. But instead our conversation stretched out, inexplicably, for almost an hour. Sheila stopped by once to silence a beeping IV pump as Marie was laughing about something, gave me a puzzled look, and left.

I'm not sure why we got along so well. Perhaps our connection wasn't really a connection at all, but merely an artifact of what I knew about her, an artificial gloss of familiarity, at least on my side. Whatever the reason, though, my visit that afternoon became a regular event. I usually stopped by in the afternoons, perhaps four or five times over the next two weeks.

In those visits we'd talk about almost anything—an exhibit at the Field Museum that I had seen but she hadn't, the relative merits of gin versus vodka for martinis, or the odd coincidence of the name of her favorite musician (Nanci Griffith) and mine (Patty Griffin). They were, I realized, about as far from typical doctor-patient conversations as I've ever strayed. But, then, I wasn't her doctor. And I hadn't even seen her in my capacity as a doctor. Her rheumatologist's initial request to me might just as easily have been handled by a social worker or a chaplain or even by the ward clerk, and I never felt as though we had a medical relationship.

It was during our second or third of these wandering conversations that, without any warning, Marie asked me what would happen to her property when she died without a will. I was a bit startled by her question, and thrown off balance, too, by the casual way in which she asked it. We had been talking about a prominent businessman who had just made a bequest to the Chicago aquarium, and although I recognized that the two topics were related, I wasn't expecting such a professional-sounding question. And I must have looked surprised.

Marie mistook my expression of surprise for doubt. She acknowledged that she didn't have much of her own, just a condo near Lincoln Park that had appreciated since she and Rosalie had bought it ten years ago. But she had inherited Rosalie's entire estate, which included some property, investments, and a considerable life insurance policy.

The answer was simple enough. I knew from taking care of another patient that her property would go to her family and that's what I told her. Unless, of course, she made out a will.

She nodded slowly, apparently unconvinced. I was puzzled, because it was a straightforward question for which she should have known the answer. She'd been a medical social worker for longer than I'd been a physician, and surely she'd fielded that question dozens of times.

But Marie didn't really want to know what would happen if she died without a will. Instead, this was a clumsy—for her—segue to another topic entirely. She wanted to know, she said, what I thought of a plan she'd been mulling over that would keep her money away from her family. And so, eventually, that was what we talked about. Not about estate law, but what she wanted to do with her estate, and why.

After much back-and-forth, she said wanted to use her money to make a point. She wanted, she said, to give her money to a prominent and very liberal charity that her parents would certainly disapprove of. "And," she said, "I want to make the bequest in my parents' names."

I couldn't help laughing. That was the way Marie was. Even when she was talking about her own death and her anger with her family—both topics sober enough to cast a pall over any conversation—she could be serious without being solemn. Besides, I still expected that Marie would recover from the infection that had brought her to the hospital this time, and so her question to me was reassuringly hypothetical.

Still, I knew Marie well enough by then to suspect that even though she was telling me what she wanted to do, and even though she was treating it lightly, she still wanted—needed—my advice. Perhaps, too, she wanted my approval. But I wasn't sure how to respond. On one hand, this was what she wanted to do, and she was free to leave her estate to whomever she wanted. On the other, I was reluctant to give even the most general advice on a question that was so far removed from medicine.

Still, the time that we had spent talking—about everything from the previous weekend's concert at the Old Town School to the ethics of keeping whales in Chicago's Shedd aquarium—hadn't been wasted. For instance, it was because of those conversations that wandered far from medicine that I knew so much about Marie's relationship with her family. More importantly, though, I also had a sense of her style. I had seen her on good days and bad days and had watched a few conversations with doctors, nurses, and visitors, and a telephone call with her mother. I felt like I was learning to anticipate what she would do or say. That knowledge made me willing to at least consider offering advice.

But what advice might I have offered? I didn't know what to say. Nor did I really understand how complicated Marie's question was. I only understood that much later. But to my credit, at least I did guess that Marie's laughing enthusiasm was not as simple as it seemed. And I thought I saw in her question a hint that perhaps she was not as confident as she appeared to be.

Revenge and Defiance

I was uncomfortable with Marie's question not only because it lay so far outside the bounds of medicine or ethics, but because our entire discussion seemed wrong somehow. Not morally or ethically wrong, but improper, as if by talking about methods of revenge and punishment, Marie was somehow flouting the unwritten conventions of dying that prescribe peace, serenity, and above all, forgiveness.

As we sat in her room talking, the example of revenge that came to me most clearly was from a book I had just read by Bruno Bettelheim, a psychiatrist and Holocaust survivor. Bettelheim tells a story that, for him, seems to embody both the horrors of the Nazis' camps and the resilience of their victims. As a group of women were being led to the gas chambers, he recalls, a Nazi officer learns that one of the women had been a professional dancer. The officer commands her to dance for him, and for the other officers. She agrees, but only to distract his attention until she deftly seizes his pistol and kills him.

I remember thinking, though, that what makes Bettelheim's example so vivid—the circumstances and the inarguable moral high ground of the woman he describes—also made it irrelevant for Marie, and indeed for most of us. How many of us will find ourselves in circumstances so extreme as to make revenge not only justified, but admirable? No, I decided, except for a very few of us, revenge isn't a worthy goal for someone like Marie who might be near the end of her life.

And so I didn't give Marie any answer at all that afternoon. Instead, I said things that I hoped would be noncommittal. I promised her I'd think about her plan.

And I did. In fact, on my way home that night, I thought of another example that prompted me to reconsider my first reaction. It was an example that bore at least a superficial resemblance to what Marie had in mind and was closer, in a way, than Bettelheim's story was.

Janusz Bardach, a plastic surgeon I knew from my time at the University of Iowa, was a remarkable survivor of the Soviet gulag. He salvaged from that experience a vast library of stories that were by turns inspiring and horrific, many of which he later described in a memoir. Newly interned prisoners, he said, would attempt to hide money and jewelry by sewing them into clothes and prison uniforms. But when it became clear that they were about to be killed, many would destroy their valuables so the camp guards, at least, would not get them. Similar stories, incidentally, come from historical accounts of the Nazi concentration camps, in which prisoners on their way to the gas chambers would throw jewelry into latrine trenches and would shred paper money to keep it from the Nazis.

There are also stories of people who have exacted a final revenge without violence. For instance, Chaim Aaron Kaplan was an elementary school principal who kept a remarkable diary of his experiences in the Warsaw Ghetto using a series of children's composition books, the only materials available to him. It is clear from Kaplan's account that he felt compelled to keep a historical record of the atrocities that he witnessed so that justice, eventually, would be served. Doing so, he says, was his "mission." Indeed, an obligation to record was perhaps one of the defining features of life during the Holocaust. Primo Levi and Elie Wiesel, for example, argued that survivors like themselves had an obligation to "bear witness" and to "testify for the future," respectively, so that the perpetrators would eventually pay for their crimes.

These are all inspiring examples of revenge—or justice—under horrendous circumstances. Together, they offer proof that it is possible to achieve some form of justice for wrongs, even when those wrongs are committed on an unprecedented scale. They offer hope, too, that even under the most impossibly grim conditions, there will be people who devote whatever time they have left to ensuring that justice is served. I don't mean to imply that whatever wrongs Marie suffered were equivalent to those in the examples I've mentioned. Certainly they represent a different scale entirely. Still, with those stories providing a frame of reference, Marie's plan began to seem more appropriate, even natural.

There are, however, no obvious parallels for all of us who can expect to die of chronic illness. We're not—most of us at least—going to die because of what a person has done to us, nor will we have opportunities for heroic revenge. However, there is one patient I took care of once whose last months took a strangely similar course.

Jaime had been in her thirties when she was diagnosed with a very rare form of bile-duct cancer that was, remarkably, detected early enough to cure. That the cancer was found at such an early stage was the result of a strange string of cancers that had afflicted other members of her immediate family and several cousins. Something, apparently, had put them all at increased risk. And so they became a family of self-described hypochondriacs, scrutinizing any anomaly—a new cough, a pang of indigestion, a worrisome mole—that might presage the arrival of the next cancer to invade their family.

Of course, they weren't hypochondriacs at all; they were simply vigilant. And their vigilance offered some degree of protection, at least for a time, allowing the early detection and cure of cancers like

Jaime's. But even the most rigorous and comprehensive cancer prevention program has limits. This is particularly true when, as in Jaime's family, there didn't seem to be an underlying pattern permitting them to focus their vigilance. So about ten years later she was sad but not particularly surprised when her vague back pain turned out to be caused by a very aggressive, and very advanced, form of pancreatic cancer. Even when pancreatic cancer is diagnosed early, survival rates are quite low. And in Jaime's case, since the tumor had spread throughout her abdomen and invaded her liver, a cure would not be possible.

The first time I met her, when she was hospitalized because of nausea that had left her dehydrated, her mother and brother were in the room as well. I had been with them for no more than ten minutes when the conversation turned to the astonishingly high incidence of cancer in their family. Like many of the doctors who had cared for them over the years, I was curious, and so I asked them what they believed was responsible.

They had a theory, they said, that the cancers were caused by the neighborhood they lived in, specifically by their proximity to the airport. When the runway whose glide path was right over their house was in use, they said, they could smell jet fuel that was unbearably strong in the back yard in the summer, and which even seeped into the house in the winter. And Jaime's mother said that, years ago, when Jaime was growing up, planes on their final approach would purge their fuel tanks, releasing jet fuel onto the Delaware River, the surrounding marshland, and onto neighborhoods nearby. She said she would go out to their car in the morning to find it covered with a thick layer of fuel residue, thick and viscous, like a layer of grease on a stove.

Over the last several years they had become increasingly convinced that the airport was the culprit. When Jaime's cancer was diagnosed at an advanced stage, proving that link became Jaime's mission. She and her mother met with local and state public health officials, with epidemiologists who specialized in studying cancer clusters, and even with several local reporters, trying to interest them in the story. All of this, they said, was in preparation for a lawsuit that they planned to bring against either the city or the airport, or perhaps both.

Hearing all this, I understood why this topic had come up so quickly in our conversation. This was a mission, or perhaps an obsession, that had consumed first Jaime's mother and then Jaime. This was how Jaime wanted to spend her time, exacting revenge on whomever or whatever was killing members of her family, and now her.

I understood her motivation, yet I wasn't entirely comfortable with it. All of this effort was taking its toll on Jaime, I thought. And it was taking time away from Jaime's husband and friends who had, at most, perhaps three or four months left to spend with her.

But when I've shared Jaime's story with medical students, for instance, I've found them wholly untroubled by such doubts. In fact, their reaction is typically one of intense admiration, even awe. What is most revealing about their reactions is that the students' attention skips so quickly ahead to consider whether they themselves would do what Jaime did. It is a given, they seem to say, that this would be a good way to use one's time. Almost dismissing that question as obvious, they turn instead to consider whether they would be able to persevere as she did. So if there's a salient lesson here for Marie, and for the rest of us, perhaps it is that acts of revenge can be truly admirable, at least when they are driven by a sense of righteousness and a desire for justice.

The Risks of Revenge

These are inspiring examples, it's true. But they're also very different, most of them, from Marie's situation. Could they really have anything to teach us about the choice that Marie was contemplating? Marie was seeking revenge for past wrongs done to her and, I suppose, to Rosalie. And it was this, more than anything, which made me uncomfortable.

The vast majority of us will die of chronic progressive illnesses that are not clearly anyone's fault. Any acts of revenge that we contemplate must necessarily be more like Marie's, directed at someone who may be guilty of many things, but not of murder. This is a crucial distinction from the stories I mentioned above.

I took care of a patient once who had been partially disabled by a workplace accident several years earlier. Mark's wife told me that he had been angry ever since the injury, believing that it was the company's fault and that their offer of a settlement was insultingly small. Mark didn't accept the settlement, but neither did he pursue a lawsuit. His wife said he seemed to be weighing his options. But when he was diagnosed with advanced lung cancer two years after his accident, she said he began to focus with renewed energy on his injury, "working himself into a state."

A few days before he began his course of radiation therapy, and without telling his wife, he hired an attorney to take his case. What followed was a race for Mark, and a grueling ordeal for his wife. Mark seemed to push harder to move the case forward, with a greater sense of urgency, because he knew his time was limited. And soon his efforts—meetings with his attorney, visits to various medical specialists—were taking up a great deal of his time. That drain on his time and energy made him angry and that anger, in turn, spurred him to even greater efforts. Throughout all of this, his wife seemed to me to be a reluctant bystander. Already distraught over the prospect of losing her husband of sixteen years, she now seemed to be losing him prematurely, and unnecessarily, to a lawsuit that could have been avoided if he had accepted the settlement that the company had offered.

I asked Mark once to help me understand why he felt such a powerful need to pursue this lawsuit. I suppose I was looking for an opening I could use to encourage him to think about how he was using his time. Perhaps, I suggested, he wanted to ensure that his wife and family would be supported financially after he died?

No, he said, it wasn't about the money. His family was already well provided for. It was simply that he had been wronged, and he was angered—infuriated—by the company's negligence. Worse, he thought their subsequent treatment of him was offensive. He wanted to teach the company that they couldn't treat employees the way they had treated him and that, if they did, they would have to pay. That is, he wanted to teach them a lesson.

Mark's situation was considerably different from Marie's, of course. And so it wasn't until much later that I made the connection between the two.

I was in Zurich for a meeting one October when the weather was unexpectedly beautiful, and days that should have been grey and overcast were warm and sunny. So one afternoon I snuck out of the meeting and spent the day on the shore of Lake Zurich, reading a book that I had found in a seedy used bookstore next to the train station. It was a memoir by Fritz Zorn (a pseudonym), who had been a Swiss professor and playwright, a self-described neurotic, and a bit of a misanthrope. Zorn blamed all his neuroses, depression, and maladjustment on his parents, and on his upbringing in a strait-laced Swiss middle class. When he was diagnosed with a fatal form of lymphoma, he decided to use his remaining time to craft a two-hundred-page intensely heartfelt if somewhat unbalanced screed against the Swiss middle class in general and his family in particular. He saw himself, he wrote with more than a little self-importance, as a cancerous cell disrupting that smug society, creating doubt and anxiety.

Perhaps I would have been more sympathetic to Zorn's condemnation if I had read it under different circumstances. But sprawled on one of the surprisingly comfortable boulders that line the lake, I was surrounded by happy Swiss families enjoying the weather. A family of four had set up a picnic on a carpet-sized scrap of beach a few feet away from me, and their children were trying, without any success, to teach me a few words of the unique species of German—Schweizerdeutsch—spoken in northern Switzerland.

My rather obvious linguistic limitations did nothing to dampen the children's enthusiasm, and I quickly became the afternoon's entertainment, for which I was generously rewarded with cheese and crackers and a few glasses of a wonderful Dézaley that their parents had chilled in the lake. These were exactly the people, I realized, whom Zorn so despised. It was a juxtaposition that made Zorn's account seems rough, unbalanced, and churlish.

After the family left, their departure punctuated with much hilarity by my final failed attempt to redeem myself by saying goodbye in German, I thought back to Mark's lawsuit against his employer. His last months had been corrupted, I thought, by the same sort of anger that Zorn's book exemplified. What struck me most vividly about both was that their anger effectively defined the way in which each would be remembered.

Mark's wife, for instance, had watched his transformation with a sort of wounded confusion as her husband disappeared into his own angry world, leaving her behind. I'm sure that his behavior during the last year of his life colored the way that she would remember him, not only, or even mostly, as a kind, solid husband and father, but also as vengeful.

Certainly, Mark's lawsuit biased the way that I remembered him. Thinking back about the last time I saw him, he seemed belittled by his anger. It was as if his furious pursuit of the lawsuit had made him smaller, less of a person.

That vengeful anger is most disturbing, I think, because of its similarity to a variety of unsavory historical examples. When plague ravaged London in 1665–66, for instance, there were widespread reports, perhaps exaggerated, of infected people, generally poor, who would throw soiled bandages into the homes of the wealthy.

This is an extreme example, certainly. Those incidents unfolded in a situation that virtually none of us will experience. Still, it has considerable value as a cautionary tale. A desire for revenge can be corrosive, producing a bitter anger that will define the way that we're remembered.

It was this anger, or something like it, that I was afraid would overtake Marie. Her plan to keep her money away from her family could lead her to concentrate on what her family had done to her, and to Rosalie. Would she arrange those insults in careful rows, obsessing over them as Mark had done his? If so, those insults, and her plan to avenge them, would eventually take over whatever time she had left.

Anger and Revenge

What ties together all these stories in my own mind is the anger that each person must have felt. Anger, that is, with no outlet, no target. Think of thousands of Londoners dying of a mysterious disease that no one understood. Or Mark or Fritz Zorn, both dying young. They had much to be angry about. And yet there was no visible tormentor, no perpetrator, against whom they could direct that anger. Perhaps Mark's lawsuit and Zorn's indictment of the middle class offered a way, however imperfect, for them to focus the anger that they felt on an obvious target. And under those circumstances many of us can expect to feel angry, yet few of us will have a natural target for that anger. And in those circumstances we'll need to create a target out of whatever materials we have at hand. At least one of my patients has managed to do that with exceptional grace.

I took care of a woman with lymphoma once who was quite young, in her late twenties, although she'd had far more experience than most people her age. Tough in a quiet, thin-lipped way, Kim had grown up in eastern Iowa in a depressed town on the banks of the Mississippi River. As local manufacturing businesses closed down or moved away, she went from job to job, finally spending a few years in the Army when she couldn't find any work at all. Her diagnosis of lymphoma was, in a way, just one more setback. And in the same way that she was angry at those businesses for moving to Mexico to find cheaper labor, she was angry at her cancer for choosing her.

But in an important way, her story was the opposite of Mark's. Whereas his anger at the unfairness of a cancer diagnosis in his forties found an outlet in a lawsuit against his employer, it seemed to me as if Kim's long-suffering anger found an outlet and a target, finally, in her cancer. Throughout the three years that I knew her, she seemed to treat her cancer as an enemy that had always been there, but which she had just recently recognized.

When her lymphoma was first diagnosed, her oncologist cleverly harnessed the energy of that anger. Survival rates for patients with Kim's type of lymphoma were very low, less than 10 percent, but he was convinced that her furious energy would help her through the most aggressive treatment regimen he could devise. And that, he thought, would give her the best possible chance of a cure.

He proved to be right. Kim did bounce back from months of harsh treatment, shrugging off complications and side effects in a quiet, workmanlike way. You could almost see her picking herself up like an unstoppable cartoon heroine, dusting herself off, and returning to the ring for another round. This went on for almost three years, until it became apparent to everyone that a cure would not be possible.

When that happened, Kim surprised her oncologist when she told him she wouldn't want to seek further treatment that would prolong her life. What she wanted, instead, was to enroll in research. Any kind of research, it didn't matter. Clinical trials testing multiple drugs, studies that involved giving blood for cancer genetics studies, and early-phase experimental studies of new drugs. She told me, and others, that she wanted to "kick that cancer's ass." Kim wasn't interested in a cure for her cancer. She had set her sights higher. She was looking for a cure for all cancer.

Much later, after she died, I learned from one of the oncology nurses that almost since the day she was diagnosed Kim had been fighting her enemy on that larger battlefield. She had, for instance, solicited donations to the American Cancer Society from many of the physicians and nurses in the outpatient cancer center where she had received most of her care. She had even collected small donations from patients in the waiting room, and surprisingly large gifts from neighbors in her small town.

You might say that Kim's diagnosis and the threat of death had made her altruistic. And I suppose that's technically true. Kim was certainly hoping that her participation in research, and the donations that she solicited, would help others. I don't mean to dismiss that aspect of the way she spent the last year of her life. But I think that those benefits were almost a side effect. Her main goal, it seemed to me, was revenge on the disease that was taking her life.

Last Impressions

Perhaps the single most important lesson of these stories for me is the range of impressions that they leave. When I think of Kim's story, for instance, I remember her as brave and tenacious. Bettelheim's dancer, too. And crusaders for justice like Jaime and Chaim Kaplan.

In a sense, I think that the wide variety of these impressions was what worried Marie and was, perhaps, what led her to ask me for my advice. How would we remember her if she prevented her family from getting her money? Would we remember her as fair and principled, firm in her beliefs about the way she and others had chosen to live their lives? Or would we think of her as mean-spirited and vindictive, a bitter woman who took her revenge in the only way she could, hurting in the process several of her nieces and nephews who might have used part of an inheritance to pay for college?

I didn't have these questions clearly in my mind when Marie asked me for advice. In fact, they didn't really crystallize for me until years later, when I spent the better part of a winter Sunday afternoon reading a file I had obtained of the last statements, spanning twenty years, of death-row inmates in Texas. As I'd expected, most included personal messages to friends and family members, words of thanks for support and encouragement, and, for many, apologies to their victims' families.

In addition, though, many were blunt expressions of outrage over the death sentence and anger at those who were carrying it out. Roy Pippin, executed in 2007, charged all those involved in his conviction ("every one of you") with murder. "Go ahead, warden," he said, "murder me." William Chappell, executed in 2002, said, "My request is that you get yourselves in church and pray for forgiveness because you are murdering me." Henry Porter, executed in 1985: "You call this justice. I call this and your society a bunch of cold-blooded murderers."

I certainly understood and even sympathized with these messages. But those angry words seemed strangely lacking in impact. Glancing blows that had no force behind them, these final words appeared to be nothing more than a continuation of lives that were angry and often violent. I knew that this wasn't necessarily true, of course, and that anger is a natural response for someone who believes he was wrongly sentenced to death, or wrongly convicted of a crime. Still, although I realized that I was being unfair, I couldn't help reading these outbursts as one more piece of evidence on the prosecution's side. This was particularly true of those transcripts that read simply, "Profanity directed at staff."

As I read through these statements, I wondered whether this was something that death-row inmates struggled with. Did they think about how to use their last statement and how to choreograph their last moments in front of witnesses and the press? Did they struggle with whether to devote their final few moments, and their final words, to anger and belligerence, or to repentance and forgiveness?

This question played out publicly at the execution of Nicholas (Nicky) Ingram, a British-American citizen who had been sentenced to death in Georgia. His lawyer, Clive Stafford Smith, recalls that Ingram had promised to spit on the warden as he was placed in the electric chair. "He wasn't willing to take part," Stafford Smith said, "in their choreography of his own death."

Ingram's execution received considerable attention in the British newspapers, and what is most salient to me in those accounts is how they focused consistently on that last act. They called him "the spitting killer"(*Sunday Express*, April 9, 1995), for instance, and "angry, defiant and contemptuous"(*Independent*, April 9, 1995). Even those newspapers that had criticized the death penalty seemed to become markedly less sympathetic, reporting that Nicky died "spitting with rage"(*Sunday Telegraph*, April 9, 1995). In reading these accounts I realized that what Nicky had envisioned as a final act of defiance against injustice was perceived by many, instead, as final proof that he was evil.

Nicky's choice offers a distilled, more potent version of the choice that Marie faced. Just as Nicky had decided that the only legitimate response to an unjust sentence was defiance, Marie believed that she could not in good conscience leave her estate to people whose views she found so reprehensible. But—and this is the important point—there was a very real risk that she would be leaving a last impression that would be an ugly and incomplete vision of who she was.

Marie

When Marie and I first talked about her will that afternoon, and how she should arrange her estate after she died, I didn't have the benefit of most of these examples. Nor was I prepared to offer any advice. But the next time I visited, she again edged the conversation around to her plan. And while I still couldn't offer an answer, at least I was better prepared to ask questions. In particular, I wanted to understand what she hoped for.

If she did leave her estate to a charity someday, perhaps in her parents' names, what did she hope that would accomplish? Did she want to hurt her family? Or teach them a lesson? Or leave them a message?

There were at least two motivations that emerged from that second conversation. First, I got the sense that Marie wanted to send her family a message. She wanted to tell them plainly that what they had done to Rosalie and her was wrong. It wasn't as though she expected them to change their thinking, as I had initially thought. No, her goals were more modest. In fact, I think she would have been content if her family had merely realized that their behavior had had negative consequences.

In addition, I think that Marie was also motivated by a sense of justice, or fairness. That is, she felt that leaving her money to her family would, somehow, reward her family's hateful behavior. And, conversely, she felt that she had an obligation not to do so. So it wasn't only that she wanted to hurt them, but also that she didn't want to give them what would amount to a gift that she felt they didn't deserve.

The following week, as I was walking back to the hospital, I thought about her analogy of an undeserved gift, and I realized that my initial uneasiness with Marie's plan had disappeared. My newfound confidence wasn't the effect of her analogy per se. Nor was it due to the other examples of revenge that I'd thought of in the interim.

It was, I think, the way that she had been able to separate her anger about her family from whatever decision she was going to make. Marie certainly did feel very strongly and was, I'm sure, also angry with her family for the way they had treated her and Rosalie. But I realized that she didn't seem to be driven by anger. Instead, she was taking care that her decision wouldn't be influenced by the worst things her mother, for instance, had done or said.

When I arrived on the ward that day, Marie's mother was there, and Sheila waved me away. So I went to see another patient and circled back to Marie's room after her mother had gone, expecting to find the wreckage of another fight. But I was surprised to find that Marie seemed no different from when I had left her the previous week, as if for once her mother's visit, usually a traumatic event, hadn't touched her. I was surprised, too, by the way that our conversation picked up where we had left off, without any preamble.

More resolved after a weekend's reflection, perhaps, or maybe galvanized by her mother's visit, Marie seemed to be even more convinced that her family shouldn't get her money. At the same time, though, she seemed to have second thoughts about the idea of giving her money to the charity she had mentioned in our first conversation. Or perhaps she had never considered that seriously. Perhaps that was just a way of getting my attention.

What bothered her most about giving her money away to an organization, she said, was that she felt she had an obligation to keep her money in her family. I must have looked surprised. True, it was a family that had treated her poorly, she said. But it was still her family.

In the end, it was Marie who came up with the solution. We had been talking about her mother's views about adoption, and how she had refused to acknowledge the young Korean girl that one of Marie's cousins had adopted. More evidence, as if any were needed, of her family's narrow views.

That example led Marie to think about her cousin, a divorced, single mother of three, who worked as a guidance counselor in an inner-city school district. She thought, too, about how she and her cousin shared many of the same values. They had never been close, mostly because Marie's mother had effectively excluded her cousin from family gatherings. But Marie knew that her cousin had a limited income and three children to support, so she would certainly appreciate the money. And Marie was sure her cousin would appreciate the gesture. So, over the weekend, Marie had begun to think about making a substantial gift to her cousin, enough at least to provide a trust fund for the children's education.

I thought Marie's was a grand plan, and I wish I could say that I was involved in making it a reality, but I wasn't. The social worker on the unit arranged for a lawyer to visit Marie to draft the will, and her plan unfolded smoothly—and quickly—without my help.

I wish that I could have listened to the phone call in which Marie told her cousin what she was planning to do. Also when Marie told her mother what she had done. I would have liked very much to have heard both conversations. But from the increasingly brief visits I had with Marie, and from what I could glean from Sheila, Marie seemed to become relaxed, almost peaceful. She seemed confident, as I was, that she had done the right thing.

As all this was being settled, Marie's infection seemed to gain ground more aggressively every day. The vertebral infection had spread locally, requiring several surgical procedures to try to de-bride—strip away—the rotten bone. After Marie had spent three weeks in the hospital, an echocardiogram to evaluate a new heart murmur found evidence of infection on two of her heart valves, and what looked like an abscess in the heart muscle next to the mitral valve. There was no point, the cardiothoracic surgeon said, in trying to put in two new heart valves that would become infected before Marie left the operating table. Faced with a stony wall of pessimism, her rheumatologist also, eventually, admitted defeat. And at some point, as all of her doctors took a step back, Marie also gave up. She finally slipped into a half-waking state that looked less like death and, oddly, more like a lingering early morning drowsiness.

SIX

Tom

Work and Habit

Tom

Most of the stories that appear in this book are unusual, colorful, and even dramatic. I've chosen to tell these stories because they're reflections of people who are remarkable in their own ways, and who have done remarkable things. But Tom did nothing unusual, re-markable, or even particularly memorable. He lived the last eight months of his life, the time that I knew him, in much the same way that he had lived his previous forty-three years—quietly, like a smooth stone sinking into a still pond.

Tom had spent his entire life, with the exception of a few months, in a small town just outside Philadelphia. He had played on the high school football team in the fall, and had worked at the community pool and at the local country club to make extra money. The summer after graduation he went to Alaska with friends to work in a salmon cannery, an epic adventure that proved to be the first and last time he traveled more than a hundred miles from home. At summer's end he came home, married his high school sweetheart, Rachel, and used his summer's earnings to put a down payment on a small house on the edge of town. That fall, Tom took a job at a local tool-manufacturing plant—the primary business in town—where he had been working ever since.

Over the next twenty-five years or so Tom and Rachel had three daughters and led lives that were almost completely uneventful. They still lived in the same house, for instance, and Tom still worked in the tool plant, as a manager now. Theirs were lives in which things didn't happen.

Three weeks before I met him, Tom had been at the plant on a Friday afternoon, working through his lunch hour to try to get caught up before the weekend. Most of the employees and other managers were either down in the plant cafeteria or at one of a line of fast-food places across the street, so Tom was alone in his glassed-in cubicle off the assembly room floor. And as he sat at his desk, reviewing productivity reports, he began to feel a tightness across his chest.

Tom was puzzled. He briefly considered, and then dismissed, the possibility that this sensation was the first hint of heart disease. He was too young for that, he decided. And besides, his heart was on the left side, and this discomfort was all over his chest. So he chewed some antacid tablets and the discomfort subsided.

But later that evening that tightness returned as he was driving out of the plant's parking lot. The pressure he felt this time was even more insistent, as if it were caused by a rope wound tightly around his chest that wouldn't let him breathe. Tom pulled off to the side of the driveway and took out his cell phone, feigning a conversation so his coworkers driving by wouldn't wonder why he was parked there on a Friday evening. That was the last thing he remembered.

Some time later a senior plant manager, who was one of the last to leave that night, found Tom slumped over the steering wheel of his car and called an ambulance. Tom was taken first to the nearest hospital and then, early the next morning, he was airlifted to the medical center at Penn. Tests found numerous pulmonary emboli—blood clots—blocking the arteries in his lungs. The result was the shortness of breath and chest tightness that Tom had tried to ignore, followed by a drop in blood pressure and a loss of consciousness as Tom's heart became unable to pump against the increased resistance.

(It's worth mentioning that I heard this story not from Tom, but from Rachel. It was a story she liked to tell to new physicians because it gave them, she thought, a good summary of Tom's attitude toward his health and his life in general. A sort of stolid optimism that no matter how grim things may look, they really couldn't be so bad.)

After a prolonged, rocky course in Penn's ICU, Tom was discharged home about two weeks later with a diagnosis of idiopathic pulmonary hypertension. All too aware that this diagnosis is usually fatal within a year, his physician at Penn referred Tom to Penn's "prehospice" service, a home care program staffed by hospice nurses with expertise in managing pain and other symptoms. My mentor Janet Abrahm had recently created the service, and it was proving to be a perfect fit for patients like Tom who were likely to die soon but who were not yet ready to think about hospice.

At that time, I was working one day a week as one of the hospice's associate medical directors, which involved caring for a small group of patients who were enrolled in hospice. In addition, I was also responsible for a few of the patients in the prehospice program. So every Wednesday afternoon I would meet with our team of nurses, social workers, chaplains, and volunteers to discuss our patients. It was at one of these meetings that I first heard about Tom from Pamela, our nurse, and Sherri, our social worker.

They had just met Tom in his home the day before and had returned to our office perplexed. Their first surprise had been that one of Tom's colleagues had brought him work to do from the plant. It was the end of the fiscal year, Tom told them, and personnel reports had to be finished and next year's department budget finalized. There were others who could have done the work, but Tom, apparently, hadn't been willing to delegate it. And so Pamela and Sherri found him sitting in his living room, tethered to an oxygen tank nestled on the sofa next to him, with a laptop in front of him, surrounded by stacks of papers and folders and file boxes.

Sherri's initial impression, she said, had been that Tom was actually much healthier than she expected. Sherri had never taken care of a patient who brought work home with him, and so Tom, she thought, didn't really "belong" in the program. He would be with them only long enough to recover from his hospitalization.

Pamela had the same impression, initially. But she also thought it was odd that Tom hadn't met them at the front door, or even in the front hallway, where they'd paused to talk with Rachel. And he'd stayed seated as they came into the living room. So Pamela, skeptical, wondered what frailty might be hidden under that veneer of industriousness.

Pamela's suspicion was confirmed a few minutes later when she noticed the pillows and blankets stacked neatly behind a well-worn recliner. So he had been sleeping in the living room, Pamela asked? It was easier, Tom said. He could avoid a laborious trip up the stairs to the bedroom, and besides, he told them, he got short of breath lying flat so he was much more comfortable sleeping in the recliner. For Pamela, this was proof that Tom was, in fact, as seriously ill as they had expected, if not more so.

But why, then, was Tom immersed in budgets and spreadsheets? Why was he surrounded by file boxes rather than by his family? This was a patient, they thought, who should be saying goodbye to his family. So why was he was filling out evaluations of assembly-line employees and estimating his department's computer budget for the coming year?

At our Wednesday team meeting, as we became tangled in these questions, we all agreed that I should visit Tom at home to try to sort them out. We needed to know whether Tom understood his diagnosis and what it meant. If he did, and this was simply how he wanted to spend his time, well, that was fine. But if not—if Tom was in denial, as Pamela and Sherri suspected—then, we agreed, we had an obligation to help him to come to terms with the likelihood that he was going to die soon. And so on a Friday afternoon, three weeks to the day after Tom's near-fatal episode in the plant parking lot, I left work early to avoid traffic and drove out of town.

Tom lived a few miles beyond the far northwest edge of Philadelphia, and as I wound my way through the increasingly diffuse neighborhoods arrayed in rings around the city, I had plenty of time to think about Pamela's and Sherri's concerns. I agreed that the work ethic they'd seen was most likely the result of denial. But it was too soon, I decided as I passed the city limits, to try to make that determination.

At forty-three, Tom was relatively young, and had been in excellent health up until the day on which he'd been given a year or less to live. So in the past three weeks he would have had to rearrange his image of himself and his future life, thinking in terms of months rather than decades. That's an enormous cognitive and emotional task that people can't accomplish in a week or two. Perhaps, then, there was no "problem" that we needed to solve at all. As I turned off the two-lane highway into Tom's neighborhood, I decided, tentatively but with a growing sense of relief, that he simply needed more time.

Tom's house was in a county that had undergone intense but haphazard development over the past twenty-five years or so. Convenience stores backed up onto horse farms that, in turn, were surrounded by subdivisions, producing jagged boundaries that separated the old and the new. Rural in Tom's grandparents' time, the land had been diced into strip malls and housing tracts, separated by thin stands of silver maple and pin oak, and a few forgotten fruit orchards. Scattered among fields and zero-lot-line houses were a few turn-of-the century homes like Tom's that had somehow escaped demolition.

I liked Tom's house immediately. At the end of a quiet street, it was a small two-story farmhouse whose gently frayed white wood-work had a sort of mature elegance next to the bright aluminum siding of its neighbors. The weathered clapboards and the old dou-ble-hung six-light windows probably wouldn't accept another coat of paint, but by some magic of aging they seemed to have become impervious to the weather. As I pulled into the cracked asphalt drive behind an immense, solid Buick, it occurred to me that Tom's house—quietly yet adamantly resisting the changes around it—offered a pretty good image of what I had heard about Tom himself.

Tom's youngest daughter met me at the door. A freshman in high school, she was dark haired, gum-snapping, and sharp-eyed, a precise replica of Rachel, whom I would meet on the way out. She led me around a clutch of giggling school friends at the kitchen table and through the swinging door into the living room.

Just as Pamela and Sherri had said he would be, Tom was sitting on an overstuffed sofa facing the living room's bay window, pillows and blankets bundled neatly on the floor next to a worn velour re-cliner in the corner. He had his feet up on two cardboard file boxes where a coffee table should have been, and had been recently, judg-ing by the four pockmarks in the deep pile carpet. And folders, dozens of them, in every conceivable color, had coalesced into piles on the sofa, on the floor, and on Tom's lap.

Tom was tall and thin in a wiry way, like a coat hanger that had been twisted into a human shape temporarily, but which has the po-tential to snap back without warning. His hair, sheared to stubble, and a mustache, only slightly longer, were the color of dried wheat. And his face was unnaturally lean, with a sharp nose and prominent cheekbones.

I noticed all this immediately, but I didn't register until much later that Tom was also surprisingly neatly dressed. A white oxford button-down shirt, a grey cardigan, and blue gabardine slacks. He looked, I realized, like he was on his way to work.

As Tom looked up and the kitchen door swung back, we both heard, distinctly, one of the girls suggesting that I didn't look old enough to be an "actual doctor." That I was more likely a medical student. Or a physician's assistant. Or something.

Tom grinned—a wide-open welcome—and waved dismissively at the kitchen door, unfurling a long arm as if he were lobbing a softball.

I thought that this was as good a place as any to start. So I began by saying I was in fact a doctor. An actual doctor. Just like Tom was an actual patient, although most of my patients didn't take their work home with them.

His grin faded, just a bit. Clearly, this was a sore subject, and probably not the best opening conversation topic. But he took it well. Rachel, he said, had been after him about working. His brother Jeremy, too, had given him a hard time.

It turned out that it was actually Jeremy's ribbing that solidified his plan to keep working. In one of their first conversations after Tom's diagnosis, Jeremy had come to visit on Tom's first day home from the hospital. He had chided Tom about the piles of paperwork that decorated the living room. Jeremy had joked that with "a serious thing like that" (Tom's illness) hanging over *his* head, *he* wouldn't be wasting time with work. Nope. He'd quit his job, rent an RV, and drive across the country. Or something. Well, he wasn't sure what he would do. But he sure wouldn't spend his time filling in boxes on spreadsheets.

Jeremy must have known then that Tom's pulmonary hypertension was a terminal diagnosis. And the certainty of Tom's approaching death, which must surely have made Jeremy uncomfortable, was perhaps impossible for Jeremy to acknowledge directly. And he also probably recognized that there was something odd about Tom's intense, myopic, focus on his work. But he wasn't sure how to bring this up without joking about it, which only solidified Tom's resolve.

Tom told me all this about Rachel's complaints, and about Jeremy's jokes. Then he was quiet. Not so much thoughtful as satisfied, as if he had answered my question.

He hadn't, of course. Not really. I had said that his use of his time seemed to me to be unusual, and he had told me, in effect, that Rachel and Jeremy thought it was unusual, too. That was hardly an answer.

But then again, maybe it was. Tom was doing what I do for many of my patients, albeit in reverse. He was validating my concern, I suppose, by telling me that others have the same concern. In the same way, for instance, I tell my patients who are afraid of experiencing severe pain that their fears are understandable, and that in fact many people feel the same way. Tom was telling me that my reaction to how he was handling his condition was natural, but not to worry, because other people had the same reaction and had learned to live with his decision. Indeed, I thought, the fact that Rachel had come to accept her husband's home office in her living room was clear proof of that. And so Tom's message to me seemed to be that if Rachel and Jeremy could accept his idiosyncrasy, then I could, too.

Still, I knew that wasn't an answer that would mollify Pamela and Sherri and the rest of the team. They had asked me for a professional opinion about whether Tom was in denial and I didn't yet have enough information to give them one. So I asked Tom about what had happened in the last several weeks, and what his doctors had told him about his prognosis. These are questions that rapidly reveal evidence of misunderstandings or denial, if it exists.

But Tom convinced me then that he had as clear a picture of his prognosis as any patient I've taken care of. For instance, he recognized that he had a serious illness that was likely to kill him in the next year. He remembered, with actuarial precision that included high- and low-confidence intervals, what his doctors had said about his prognosis. He even remembered that his cardiologist and his ICU physician had given him slightly different survival estimates. However, he smiled, even though the cardiologist's estimate seemed unshakably confident, he had given two very different estimates in different conversations a day or two apart. So Tom tended to believe the ICU physician. Tom told me all of this, filling in numbers and probabilities along the way. Tom, it was clear, was not in denial.

So why, then, was he spending his time—which he knew was very limited—on budgets and spreadsheets? I didn't have an answer to that question yet, and I probably wouldn't find one, at least on that visit. It was getting late, and the sky framed by the bay window next to us had grown dark. Tom's family was congregating in the kitchen, and I felt as though I were holding him hostage. Besides, Tom was obviously tired. He was speaking more slowly and deliberately, choosing words carefully and occasionally losing his place in the conversation. And he'd lost the animation that I'd seen an hour before.

So I realized I wouldn't leave with an explanation for the piles of paperwork all around us. Still, I told myself, as long as he understood that he did not have much time left, however he chose to spend that time was up to him. More than that, it seemed inappropriate, or at least inappropriately intrusive, for me to judge that choice.

As I drove back down the winding county highway that connected Tom's town with the Philadelphia city streets, my old truck's yellow headlights groped weakly along the road just a few yards ahead. Normally that poor visibility was frustrating, but that night I found the lack of visibility vaguely comforting. A sort of enforced denial, since I'd have no advance notice of the raccoon, or deer, or tree I was about to hit. And so although this sort of drive would usually have taken all my attention, that night I found myself thinking not of the deer that might materialize a few feet in front of me but instead of that image of Tom in his living room. I could still see him sitting there, alone, hunched over a spreadsheet, adding, subtracting, and editing. It seemed familiar, somehow. A Dickens novel, maybe.

But as I reached the well-lit streets of Chestnut Hill at the edge of the city, I realized that the echo I heard didn't come from a novel. What seemed so familiar about Tom's story was that he reminded me of myself. As clearly as I could see Tom, I could visualize myself, faced with a terminal diagnosis, doing exactly the same thing. Finishing a last paper or two. And wrapping up the data analysis for a study so a colleague could write it up. And it was this connection, more than anything Tom had said to me, that made me want to defend his choice.

Why shouldn't he keep working, I thought, if that's what he wanted to do? It's true that none of our other patients continued to work with anywhere near the tenacity that Tom had demonstrated. But Pamela, Sherri, and I were accustomed to taking care of patients with substantial physical frailty or cognitive impairment. That is, the vast majority of our patients couldn't work. But Tom could, and so he did. And not only did he continue to work, but, as I learned later, he also adhered to the schedules and customs of work. In fact, he'd dressed that morning just as he would have a month earlier, and he tried to keep the same work hours that he would have kept in the office.

Still, to say that Tom kept working because he could was hardly a satisfying explanation, particularly since Tom's was a job that, at least from my perspective, had the intellectual appeal of assembly-line work. Should he have continued to work? Was that really the right choice for him? And would it be, someday, the right one for me?

These became the most compelling questions as I drove along the Schuylkill Expressway toward the city, against rush-hour traffic. Rather than go home to an empty house and barren refrigerator, I had decided earlier in the day that I would go back to my office at Penn and work late that night, picking up dinner from one of the street vendors who stayed open for people like me. And so my truck and I were rumbling in toward the city, catching glimpses occasionally of faces that appeared out of the snarl of traffic in the westbound lanes. They were all, I imagined, returning to homes, husbands, wives, families, and refrigerators that held more than a few shriveled limes and a loaf of fuzzy bread. As I thought about Tom, and about the grant I had to finish writing that night, there didn't seem to be much distance between us. If he was wasting his time, I realized, then perhaps I was, too.

Denial

I was convinced that Tom wasn't in denial, but at our team meeting the following week I faced a skeptical audience. Pamela, in particular, was unconvinced. How else could we explain why Tom was spending what would be his final months surrounded by files and forms? This was the worst part of being a nurse, she thought, and she couldn't believe that anyone as intelligent and personable as Tom could devote his limited time to something that she so disliked.

In Tom's defense I pointed out that he wasn't seeking further treatment. Tom recognized that he had reached the limits of what medicine could do for him. I didn't think that someone could agree that treatment was futile yet still cling, somehow, to the belief that he could look forward to a long life. That logic was met with a few moments of what I flattered myself was awed silence.

But Pamela wasn't satisfied. She admitted that Tom didn't want further treatment. But some people in denial might want treatment, she said, and others might not. Just as a patient might have an illness without a symptom, maybe Tom was in denial without this particular "symptom."

Pamela, Sherri, and the rest of the team turned to look at me. Clearly, I was going to have to work harder to convince this group. So we interrupted the team meeting and I gave an impromptu lecture on denial.

It's actually easier to understand denial, I said, or at least to define it, by thinking about its opposite. That is, it helps to think instead about what it takes for people to be able to make decisions. We usually say that people can make decisions—that they have decision-making capacity—if they can do three things.

First, they need to be able to understand the facts related to a decision. I used hospice enrollment as an example, since this was a decision that everyone in the room was familiar with. In order to have the capacity to make a decision about hospice enrollment, a patient would need to be able to understand what hospice is. He would also need to understand the advantages and disadvantages of enrolling. For instance, he'd need to know about the hospice services that he'd receive, and also that he'd have to forgo some treatments in order to enroll.

Second, he would need to be able to weigh those advantages and disadvantages. For instance, he'd need to be able to add up the advantages of enrolling in hospice and compare them with disadvantages of doing so. And he'd need to be able to say why enrolling in hospice is or isn't the best choice for him.

Third, he would need to be able to recognize that all of these facts apply to him. This aspect of decision-making capacity, called "appreciation," is a key element of decision-making capacity because it ensures that a person like Tom recognizes that his decision will affect him. And the opposite of appreciation, I said—denial—is what we were concerned about in Tom's case.

To emphasize the importance of appreciation and denial, I told the team about an older African-American woman with diabetes I had seen in medical school, while I was on the infectious disease consult service. About a year before her hospitalization, a stroke had left Barbara with impaired speech and with limited movement of one side of her body. A few weeks before her hospitalization, she had developed an infection in her "good" foot, the one unaffected by her stroke.

Barbara's diabetes had produced extensive nerve damage, and so her infection didn't cause any pain, even as it spread into the bones of her heel and up through the muscles in her calf. It wasn't until she became confused, with high fevers, that her granddaughter grew concerned and brought her to the emergency room. By the time she arrived, the infection had engulfed Barbara's right leg, spreading rapidly between planes of muscle. The infectious-disease doctor who ran the consult service that month had been told that this was a routine infection and so he sent me, as the medical student, to see the patient first.

Initially, I had the same impression, until the resident in the emergency room pointed out an X-ray finding that should have been obvious to me, if I hadn't been in such a hurry to wrap up a "routine" case. On a second look, clearly visible, were thin dark bands between planes of muscle that were a classic sign of a gas-producing bacterial infection—"gas gangrene"—an infection that is so aggressive that its advance through tissue can be measured hour by hour. Antibiotics typically have no effect and the only hope of a cure lies in an emergency amputation.

But when the resident and I went in to meet her, Barbara stolidly refused to agree to surgery to amputate her leg. The resident and I were confused at first, noting her clumsy speech and thinking—hoping—that perhaps we had misheard her. But she understood everything we told her. She understood, for instance, everything I've just written about gangrene, what causes it, and what the only treatment is.

Barbara could also weigh the risks and benefits of surgery rationally. That is, she could tell us that if she had a terrible infection like that in her leg, she would certainly agree to surgery, if doing so would save her life. This gave us ample evidence of her reasoning ability.

I should note, too, that someone's reasoning ability doesn't depend on the answer they give. For instance, Barbara might have told us that, up until that point, her good leg had allowed her to be relatively independent, at least in cooking and cleaning and taking care of her house. But the amputation would confine her to a wheel-chair, which would have required her to move in with her daughter, or into a nursing home. If she had said this, and explained that the trade-off we were proposing—amputation in exchange for her life—was unacceptable to her, that would also have demonstrated evidence of her ability to reason.

And so Barbara understood everything we told her, and she was able to say why surgery for gangrene was really the only option. So why, we asked her, didn't she want surgery?

Now it was her turn to be surprised. She didn't understand what this discussion had to do with her, she said. It had been very interesting, and she appreciated our taking the time to visit, but *she* didn't have gangrene. The resident and I sat there stunned for a few moments, glancing at each other to confirm, for the second time in a few minutes, that we had heard correctly.

Barbara didn't want surgery, apparently, because she didn't believe she had gangrene. In fact, she didn't believe anything was wrong with her at all. She had a fever that was probably the flu. The flu was going around, she said. Did we know that? She had been feeling "out of sorts" for the last two weeks, she told us, that's all this was. We must have appeared skeptical, because she rattled off a list of symptoms of infection that she hadn't had, or hadn't been aware of, such as fever, swelling, and pain.

The pièce de résistance, in Barbara's mind, was that she hadn't had any pain, which we knew was because her diabetic neuropathy had eliminated most sensation in her feet. But for her, this was clear evidence, as if any were needed, that this couldn't possibly be gangrene. Nor was she convinced by our interpretation that she couldn't feel pain because of her diabetes. If this infection were really as severe as we said it was—severe enough to require amputation—then surely it should hurt just a little bit? So, she concluded triumphantly, there's really no chance that this is the sort of infection that you're talking about.

Barbara could understand her situation and could even weigh the risks and benefits of surgery, but she couldn't appreciate how all of that information applied to her. And because of that, it was virtually impossible for us to engage her in further discussion. She was pleasant and polite, but she honestly didn't believe that what we were talking about, with increasing exasperation, had anything to do with her.

I wish I could say that we were able to convince her otherwise. But overcoming denial, I've since learned, is enormously difficult. After several hours of discussion, in which I was only partly involved, it was Barbara's granddaughter who was able to convince her, finally, to agree to surgery. Even that, though, was too late. In the time from our first meeting until surgery later that afternoon, the infection had spread too far to control and she died in the surgical intensive care unit the next day.

There are many other patients I've taken care of whose ability to make decisions was impaired by denial. I could have used any one of these examples. But I chose Barbara's because it was extreme and therefore offered a clear illustration. And I also wanted to make the point to the team that, whatever was going on in Tom's head, it wasn't denial. Indeed, when viewed next to Barbara's example, Tom's behavior seemed eminently sensible. At least, that's what I hoped the team would think.

I'm not sure my minilecture on decision-making capacity entirely satisfied them. Pamela, certainly, was still skeptical. She was still unable to imagine that Tom could devote his time to budgets and paperwork if he knew that he had only months to live. Still, we had other patients to talk about. And besides, we decided, Tom's problem, if in fact it was a problem, seemed to be more disturbing to us than it was to him, or even to his family. So as long as we were convinced that Tom wasn't in denial, we were comfortable that we had done what we could, at least for now.

Motivations

Our team had come to a consensus that we could all live with, and we moved on to review our other patients. But I continued to think about Tom's motivations, as I suspect Pamela and Sherri and others did as well. It was easy enough to declare that Tom wasn't in denial. But that resolution wasn't a very comfortable one.

In fact, it reminded me of a bizarre scene I witnessed once as a medical student. An older man had come to the emergency room alone, complaining of chest pain that sounded like "typical" pain caused by coronary artery disease. The man was alone, anxious, and obviously frightened by the pain, and by thoughts of what might be causing it. After a rapid but thorough workup that revealed no evidence of heart disease, an officious resident I hadn't seen before ducked through the curtain surrounding the man's bed and told him firmly that there was nothing wrong and that he could go. The resident ducked back out as quickly as he had come, leaving my patient looking at me in confusion, with just as much anxiety as he had shown moments before—even more, perhaps, now that he was being sent away without a diagnosis. In the same way, I thought, we had ruled out the worst possible explanation for Tom's behavior—that he was in denial—but we were no closer to understanding that behavior than we had been the previous week.

What would have made Tom behave the way he did, if he wasn't in denial? What could explain the hours spent hunched over a laptop, and the mountains of files that surrounded him? It wasn't as though he were writing a book, or wrapping up an academic career, which were things that I could imagine myself doing if faced with a fatal diagnosis. No, his focus on trivial, administrative work didn't make sense to me. Just as I would have liked to have been able to offer a diagnosis and a plan to my patient with chest pain in the emergency room that night, I wanted some sort of "diagnosis" that would explain Tom's choices. I hoped for a diagnosis that would tell us how we could help him to choose more wisely, but I would have been content with one that gave us permission to simply leave him alone.

Distraction

One possible explanation of Tom's behavior that I considered was that his work was simply a distraction from the illness that he was facing. He had heard an enormous amount of bad news in the past several weeks. Too much, really, to assimilate fully. Perhaps he was fully aware of his situation, but he just didn't want to think about it. Faced with long days at home, too short of breath and too fatigued even to climb the stairs to his bedroom every night, how could he take his mind off the illness that would kill him? His work, maybe, was simply the most readily accessible means of distraction.

Indeed, this would probably be true for many of us, particularly those of us whose work involves writing. When she was diagnosed with metastatic breast cancer, the *Washington Post* writer Natalie Spingarn would actively search for distractions in her work. She called hers "the workaholic road." Whenever she found herself thinking obsessively about her cancer and her prognosis, she said, she would turn to her next column. Or she'd seek out a new writing assignment or look for another consultant job. It wasn't as if Spingarn was ignoring her illness. In fact, for several years her column focused on cancer and its treatment. Yet the process and mechanics of writing—of work—offered distraction and distance.

But for Spingarn, and probably for Tom as well, I think the distraction of work came with a catch. The respite that work seemed to offer both of them depended entirely on their jobs and on their ability to retain those jobs. If Spingarn gave up her column, she would have given up not only her identity and livelihood, but also the source of distraction in which she found the most comfort. Tom, too, must have realized that if he slowed down he might be put on sick leave or laid off. And if that happened, he would have to look elsewhere for a source of distraction. So for both Spingarn and Tom, and perhaps for many of us, the distraction of work is tenuous, offering comfort but requiring considerable energy to maintain.

I realize, of course, that to compare Tom's work with that of a writer is a little misleading. Whereas Spingarn's source of distraction was in the creativity of writing, Tom must have found his in the seemingly endless columns and figures in the piles of paperwork that surrounded him. So it seemed to me that the distraction—if that's what it was—that Tom had found was a more elemental kind. It was almost as if he wanted to keep his mind busy, I thought.

Tom's form of distraction seemed less like Spingarn's and closer to that of Ron Flory and Tom Wilkinson, two miners trapped by a fire in Idaho's Sunshine silver mine, almost a mile below the surface. On their fourth day underground, the two men became convinced that they had been forgotten and began to talk about how their wives would spend their life insurance payments. To push those sorts of thoughts out of their minds, they devised an intricate series of tasks, like making a square braid out of blasting wire. Just as a difficult puzzle might, these tasks absorbed the men's attention, constraining their wandering thoughts and fears. Perhaps Tom had found a similar sort of distraction in the columns of figures and the intensity of concentration that they required.

Familiarity and Habit

Although I thought it was possible that the spreadsheets with which Tom had surrounded himself offered the relief of distraction, I also recognized that there were other plausible explanations. If some of us continue to follow the paths of our everyday lives—child care, housekeeping, jobs—because of the distraction that those activities offer, others, I think, follow those paths simply out of familiarity and habit. These are the activities that take up most of our time when we're well, so the force of those habits isn't reduced by a terminal diagnosis.

Indeed, I've been surprised by how often people who are nearing the end of their lives seem to fight to preserve the routines and habits that I would be glad to jettison. One of the strangest examples of this odd perseverance comes from the memoir of Peter Noll, a Swiss law professor who refused treatment for bladder cancer and then kept a diary that described in vivid detail that last year of his life. At first, Noll was optimistic about the way that his imminent death would force him to make better choices about how to spend his time. But he soon found that he was unwilling to give up tasks like reading students' dissertations, a process that Noll himself described as not unlike being forced to walk in the rain without a raincoat. His descriptions of interminable faculty meetings and internecine academic power struggles were equally vivid, and no less mind-numbing.

The irony, of course, is that Noll could easily have refused these responsibilities. In the form of his illness, Noll had been handed a ready-made and ironclad excuse for avoiding almost any obligation. What better justification for begging off a faculty meeting or committee than one's imminent death? So why, then, did Noll continue dragging himself through endless piles of mediocre dissertations?

Denial and distraction don't provide an explanation. Noll was aggressively, almost abrasively vocal about his illness. In fact, he wanted his last months to serve as a very visible reminder to others of their own mortality. Certainly, he made no effort to hide his illness or to present himself as anything other then terminally ill.

Instead, I think the explanation that fits best in Noll's case, and perhaps to some degree in Tom's, is that his despised dissertations and faculty meetings, like Tom's spreadsheets, were a habit that was both comfortable and comforting. His days had always been defined by the demands of faculty meetings, office hours, exams, and dissertations. And just as the hanging loops on a subway car give passengers a firm anchor, converting random twists and turns into a gentle swaying, the mundane activities of everyday life impose a more gentle and predictable rhythm on the chaos of life with a serious illness.

To some degree, too, I suspect that Noll and Tom clung to these routines because of the relationships they brought. That is, these routines are also the trusses and cables that hold relationships together. Think for a moment of the interactions we have with dozens of people every day. Take away those routines and those relationships, too, fall apart. Some of those relationships can be rather close, like the semifriendships of the workplace or with your daughter's swimming coach. Others are more distant, like the Korean lady who owns a dry-cleaning business across the street from my office. But they're all relationships that provide comforting reminders that we're still here.

Financial Security

Although I thought quite a bit about Tom's dedication to his work, and about what might be motivating him, I missed what was perhaps the most obvious explanation. Yet I can at least find some comfort in the fact that almost everyone else on the team did too. It was our social-work intern who asked us at a subsequent Wednesday meeting whether, perhaps, Tom might be working because he had to?

Rachel worked only part time, the intern pointed out. They had one daughter attending college and two more who probably would be soon. Perhaps they couldn't afford to lose Tom's income? And they were almost certainly all relying on Tom's health insurance, which was available only though his job.

She was correct to think about this, of course, and the rest of us were embarrassed to have missed it. In fact, the financial burdens of serious illness on patients and families can be substantial. For instance, several studies have found that the combination of a patient's lost employment and increased health-related expenditures can tip a family toward bankruptcy. Moreover, as a patient's family members begin to take on the increasing burdens of caregiving, they may need to sharply reduce their schedule of work outside the home, often giving up a job entirely. The result is that a family's financial stability is often threatened, leaving them with considerable debts after the patient has died.

So perhaps Tom needed to keep working. Or perhaps—and this amounts to much the same thing—Tom merely believed that he had to keep working. Tom and his apparent obsession with work reminded me more than a little of Archie Hanlan, who had been a professor of social work at the University of Pennsylvania before I joined the faculty. Hanlan had just taken a teaching position at Penn when he was diagnosed with amyotrophic lateral sclerosis (ALS), also known as Lou Gehrig's disease, a progressive neurological disease that gradually eroded his ability to climb stairs, to walk, and finally to speak. Throughout his illness, and despite the relentless progression of his disease, Hanlan continued, obstinately, to work.

In his memoir he concedes that there were many reasons he clung to his work. It kept him busy, for instance. And it made him feel useful. But overshadowing all of these motivations was a fear that he would leave his family destitute. He knew that this was not an acute concern and that they would be adequately supported, but he was compelled to keep working by a fear that to do otherwise would be to fail as a provider. And so he kept teaching. And he adhered closely to the rituals and routines of academic life—leading seminars, grading papers, attending interminable faculty meetings— far past the point at which most people would have quit.

But Tom's work ethic apparently wasn't due to financial concerns. Our social work intern determined that Tom and Rachel were reasonably well off, and Tom's employer offered a very generous life insurance policy. So there would be enough to support all three of their daughters through college.

A Sense of Identity

Some of us, at least, will continue to follow the same routine—including work—because that routine defines who we are, or at least who we'd like to be. But as I considered various explanations for Tom's apparent dedication to his work, this was one that I rejected almost immediately. Perhaps influenced by Pamela's dismissive comments about "paperwork," and probably by my own preconceptions of Tom's work, I couldn't imagine that his identity might be tied to a job like his.

So what sort of person would be compelled by his sense of his identity to continue working? Here I have to admit that my assessment was more than a little biased. Such a person would be a writer, a researcher, a thinker, naturally. It would be someone, I thought—untroubled by modesty—like me.

But a month or two after I met Tom, I took care of Ella, whose story made me realize, much later than I should have, that my patients are able to find an identity in virtually any work. Ella came from a very large Italian family in South Philadelphia, in the heart of Little Italy. Her parents had come to Philadelphia as teenagers, just married, along with several cousins from their village in northern Italy. She could count dozens of relatives in the neighborhood, and frequently did, as if to reassure herself that they were still there. And often, it seemed, Ella's kitchen was the center of that extended family. Whenever one of our team went to visit her, they'd find a small crowd of people in the kitchen and spilling out onto the front porch when the weather was nice. Ella had always been respected and feared in the neighborhood for her vigorous energy, accompanied by an indomitable confidence. 'Ispettore,' the inspector, everyone called her.

But by the time I met Ella, she had lost most of her formidable abilities. She was no longer able to cook, for instance, and she couldn't even shop in the neighborhood without help. A month or two before she enrolled in hospice, Ella had become too weak to bake the daily offering of pasticciotti—custard-filled cream puffs. Instead, she would send one of her grandchildren down the street to Isgro's to buy a box of cannoli.

Finally, the routine that she clung to more vigorously than all the others, though, was her cleaning. Ella would wake up at five o'clock every morning and start the coffee percolating. She would take out her brooms and mops and dust rags, and prepare her furniture polish and an eye-watering ammoniac floor cleaner. Pausing for a few sips of a powerful brew that might well have done double duty as a cleaning product, she would set about disinfecting her small row house, readying it for another day of visitors. I imagined that this had been her routine ever since she moved into the house in which she would live for sixty years with her husband and family, and finally, alone.

But soon after we met her, it was obvious that this was one more routine that Ella was going to have to give up. Just walking down the narrow stairs from her bedroom was an ordeal for her, and she no longer had the strength or the balance to wield a mop with the vigor that her standards of cleanliness demanded. Yet there were family and neighbors stopping by. More, now, than there ever had been. Ella couldn't bear to think that old Mrs. Tommasini would see the mud tracks that the youngest Marretti boy's work boots had left on the kitchen floor the evening before. No, her house had to be perfect even if—or perhaps because—her health was not.

The daily routine of cleaning that is for most of us a chore to be avoided was a deep-seated part of who Ella was and how she wanted to be seen. This work was as intricately tied to her identity as, say, a writer's might be. And since then, once I began looking for them, I've seen many examples of people who continue to work because that work defines who they are: a physician colleague with incurable lymphoma, for instance, who continued to work through a course of palliative chemotherapy; or an administrator in a state agency who continued to work despite a progressive autoimmune disease; or a taxi driver I met once in Syracuse who stayed on the job despite advanced heart failure. All of these people told me that they weren't working because they needed the money—the social-work intern taking care of Tom taught me to ask this question—but because they felt they had to in order to stay whole, and in order to main their self-respect.

At the time, though, I couldn't reconcile this explanation with what I knew about Tom. No matter how I looked at Tom's life and his job, I couldn't quite imagine Tom's devotion to his work as an expression of who he was. Nor could Pamela or Sherri or other members of the team.

Hidden Last Acts

Tom's condition improved over the next few weeks, surprising us and, I think, Tom himself. He was discharged from our program when he no longer needed nursing care, an event that was bittersweet because we were pleased that he was doing well and sad to see him go. But Pamela stayed in touch with Rachel, convinced that we would be seeing Tom again.

Over the next month or so, Pamela told us that Tom continued to improve, even going to work a couple of days every week. But to make those trips Tom had to mortgage most of his remaining strength, as Rachel saw it, reversing what had been a positive trend and setting him back close to where he had been when he was discharged from the hospital. It was at that point, I think, that Rachel's and Pamela's phone calls became more frequent. They were both worried, in different ways, that Tom was pushing himself too hard. And so Pamela began bringing the latest phone calls to our team meetings.

But Tom wasn't our patient, and these updates made me feel uncomfortably like a voyeur. Also, although I didn't begrudge the time we devoted to discussing his case, I didn't think we were helping him, or Rachel. And talking about him in absentia seemed both incomplete and unfair, because we were hearing only from Rachel, via Pamela, both of whom had their own strong views about Tom's work ethic.

Still, Pamela continued to bring updates to our Wednesday meetings. Perhaps she sensed something about Tom that I hadn't recognized, or perhaps she had become so close to Rachel that she had trouble disengaging. Whatever the reason, Tom's deviation from the usual glide path of a hospice patient was more jarring to Pamela than it was to us. She was clearly struggling to understand Tom's obsession with work and to decide what help, if any, she should offer.

I wish I could say that I found a way to make sense of Tom's choices. Instead, it was Belinda, our volunteer coordinator, who placed a frame around Tom's behavior that helped Pamela and the rest of us to see what our role should be. Her tentative suggestion at one team meeting was that maybe we were looking at Tom's case backward.

We were spending too much time—she tapped her watch—thinking and talking about what we thought Tom shouldn't be doing. But there wasn't much point in talking about what Tom shouldn't do, was there? He'd already shown that he would do what he wanted. Wasn't the real question, she asked, whether there was anything that Tom should be doing that he wasn't?

Because bridge-program patients like Tom didn't receive volunteer services, Belinda had never met him, and she knew less about him than anyone else around the table. But the silence that settled on the group suggested, to me at least, that Belinda had got it right. Rather than wasting our time, and Rachel's, talking about what Tom shouldn't be doing, why didn't we focus on things that we thought he could be doing with whatever time he had left?

So did we know whether Tom had completed a will, I asked? Silence around the table. Maybe he had written letters to his wife or children? More silence. It quickly became obvious that we didn't know what, if anything, Tom had done without our knowledge, and perhaps without Rachel's.

In fact, as I've learned from other patients, these sorts of hidden last acts are really quite common. One man I took care of a year or two later was steadfastly resistant to hospice's counseling efforts and their offers of spiritual support. He knew that he was dying, but he didn't want to be reminded of that fact every day. He was polite but stubborn. There was to be no talk of death, no discussion of memorial services, no life review.

And so I was surprised, later, when his daughter opened the thick manila envelope she found in the drawer of his bedside table. I'd seen it before, partially concealed by blankets or propped against the water carafe next to his bed. I had assumed that it contained medical records, or perhaps hospital bills or prescriptions. In fact, his daughter said, it held all, or most, of the things that he had rejected when the hospice social worker suggested them: letters to his daughters, postcards for his grandchildren, and succinct instructions for a memorial service. He had been doing everything we had suggested, but quietly, unobtrusively, and without our help.

Sometimes these hidden last acts are tiny, noticed only by a few. One of my favorite examples comes not from one of my patients but from *Gain*, a wonderful novel by Richard Powers. In it, the main character dies slowly and painfully of ovarian cancer. Her story, actually, is one small part of the narrative, which tracks the growth to dominance of a large pharmaceutical and manufacturing firm. Against that backdrop of the hard practicalities of manufacturing, chemicals, and waste, it's perhaps fitting that her hidden last act was a pragmatic one. Unknown to her family, she scatters Post-it notes around the house with cryptic but decipherable instructions—when to plant the bulbs in the spring, for instance, and how long to defrost the pot roast before placing it in the oven.

I sometimes use this example in a joking way with my patients. What will your family do after you're gone, I ask? Is there anything that they'll want to know, or that they'll need to know? Were you planning on leaving notes scattered around the house? Absurd yet oddly practical, the comic notion of leaving notes around the house often galvanizes my patients into making some sort of plan for the future.

In fact, many make small, often hidden plans, which anticipate their deaths. None of them has used Post-it notes, as far as I know, but they've made quiet arrangements regarding money, debts, wills, and the like. These examples aren't obvious, often, because they blend into the day-to-day activities in which we're all engaged. Of course, she arranged her will, we might say, but she didn't do anything else.

But in a sense, even these practical arrangements serve as a foundation for others. At the very least, they discharge obligations and provide us with a sense of peace that, often, we need in order to turn our attention to other things. I'm thinking, for instance, of one miner in the 1958 Springhill mining disaster in Nova Scotia who was focused—obsessed, really—with $1.40 he still owed for his car's radiator hose. He told two sociologists who studied the miners' responses after the accident that he was worried about leaving that debt, and about what people would think of him. Those sociologists interpreted the miner's focus as a kind of distraction, which I suppose could have been true. But it seems equally possible to me that he simply needed to find some way to settle that debt before he could think about other things. And I like to think that once he wrote a note to his wife that defined his debt and asked her to pay it, then he was able to think about what else he needed to say to her.

Even the most mundane, pedestrian last acts can succeed rather grandly in reminding friends and family of who we were. In what is one of the most moving yet genuinely funny descriptions of someone's last days, the writer Jonathan Raban recounts interrupting a sailing voyage along Alaska's Northwest Passage to attend to his father as he was dying of cancer in the U.K. For virtually all of his illness, he says, his father had preserved the stiff upper lip right and proper to an Anglican priest. He seemed to stride through his last days with a regimental resolution, chin up and eyes forward.

And yet, after his father died, Raban found a ten-page set of detailed instructions that included, among other things, instructions for disposal of his remains (cremation); disposal of his ashes (to be scattered and emphatically *not* kept on a mantel); and potential locations for disposal of his ashes (several possibilities, with instructions to make the trip into a weekend holiday). Other chattering suggestions abound, including funeral arrangements, instructions for a reception, and advice for guest parking.

As I read Raban's description, I was struck that these were not simply practical instructions, although that was, of course, their intended purpose. In the few paragraphs that Raban reproduces, oddly, I felt I got a better sense of his father's playfully stalwart good humor than I had from all of Raban's recollections. One gets the sense that Raban did, too, and he let those instructions serve as the last word on his father's life.

This, for me, is one of the best examples of the impact that these sorts of hidden last acts can have. Not in their stated purpose—settling a debt, arranging finances, providing instructions for a memorial service—but in the layers that surround each. These are the layers that reminded Raban's family, for instance, that his father was not just stoic, but also warm, funny, and generous. And also that he was just a bit more prescient, perhaps, than they had imagined.

Tom

None of us was surprised when Marti, our office manager, told us that Tom was coming back to us, this time as a hospice patient. Pamela went out to see him that afternoon expecting, I think, to find the same patient that she had last seen over a month before. But she was surprised by how much Tom had changed. So surprised, in fact, that she called me from her car, idling a block or two from Tom's house.

She told me, first, that all of the boxes and piles of folders were gone. Cleaned out, Rachel had told her, by a "crew" from the plant. Pamela said this with more than a little admiration, as perhaps Rachel had as well. That Tom had managed, through sheer stubbornness, to amass so many boxes and files had been eminently frustrating. But all of that was forgotten, apparently, now that he had enrolled in hospice. Now those piles were an achievement worthy of considerable pride, and perhaps a little amusement.

The second thing Pamela noticed, she said, was how weak Tom had become. Weak, and vulnerable, too, with very little of the self-contained energy that had driven him only a few months earlier. Tom was acting, finally, like a hospice patient.

Perhaps emboldened by Tom's decline, which made him more like a typical patient, or perhaps relieved by the disappearance of the file boxes, Pamela found the nerve to ask Tom why he had spent so much of his time working. Pamela told me that Tom seemed surprised by the question. Maybe he had forgotten just how much of an issue his work had been for Rachel. Or perhaps Rachel had continued to voice her concerns to Pamela privately but had stopped sharing them with Tom, knowing that he wouldn't listen. Whatever the reason, Pamela said that she seemed to have caught Tom unawares, as if she had asked about a long-forgotten misdemeanor committed in his youth.

Pamela said that Tom gave her two answers, more or less. First, he said that even when he first met us, surrounded by evidence of his work, that hadn't been the only thing on his mind. In fact, he had been organizing and planning. For instance, he'd found a shoe-box full of snapshots from his summer spent at the cannery in Alaska, and had collected them in a photo album. And he had organized the family's financial records and had prepared their taxes in readiness for the upcoming April deadline.

I realized then that we really hadn't known what was in all of those boxes and folders. We had simply assumed that they were all work-related. In any case, Belinda had been right. We should have focused more on precisely what Tom had been doing.

But Pamela is nothing if not persistent, and she pursued the question. Why had he continued to work? She understood that he had been using some of his time for other projects. But why did he let work take up any of his time?

Pamela told Tom that the team was worried that he was in denial, but Tom seemed puzzled. No, of course not, he told her. He knew his was a "bad news diagnosis" as soon as he heard it. Why else would he have been getting his family's finances in order?

Pamela paused. She was waiting, I thought, for me to ask the obvious question, which I did. So why had Tom spent so much time on his work? But Pamela hadn't been waiting for my question. I think that she was still trying to sort out what Tom had told her, and trying to reconcile that with whatever narrative she had been carrying around with her for the last few months.

Tom, she believed, had kept working because that was the kind of person he was. Pamela spoke more quickly now, enthusiastic now because she thought she finally understood what had driven Tom. It wasn't his job that he identified with, she said. Being a middle manager at a manufacturing plant wasn't part of his identity. And he certainly wasn't invested in his actual work. The spreadsheets and budgets and personnel reports were as dull to him, I think, as Pamela's admission forms were to her.

Instead, Pamela said, she thought that Tom was a hard worker. That was how he viewed himself. His identity, if that's what it was, was that of a hard worker, someone who always got the job done. That was the sense of identity that defined him, and that's the identity that motivated him to surround himself with folders and boxes when other people, perhaps, would have chosen to surround themselves with friends and family.

If Pamela was correct—and I think she was—then we had all missed the point of Tom's efforts to stay on the job long after others would have quit. It wasn't the familiarity his job offered, or the income it provided. It wasn't that Tom was committed to his job, or even that he loved it, although I supposed he liked it well enough.

He wasn't invested in his job, or even the day-to-day work. What he identified with, and what kept him at work to everyone's consternation, was the image of someone who was dependable and solid. That's who he was, and that's how he wanted to be remembered by his coworkers, his friends, and his family.

I was hearing all of this through Pamela, of course, so there were questions I would like to have been able to ask Tom. For instance, I wondered whether he regretted the time he spent with those spreadsheets rather than with his family. Did he feel that his identity as a dependable worker took time away from other things? Should we, perhaps, have pushed him harder to stop working? Or could we have at least given him permission to stop working? I would have wanted to ask these questions and more. But I didn't have a chance to ask. Tom died in his sleep, at home, two weeks later.

Perhaps that's just as well. I think that these sorts of questions wouldn't have helped Tom. Throughout the time that we knew him, he had a better sense of his priorities than we'd ever had. And he had, I think, been on the right track all along.

SEVEN

Lacy

Memories and Legacies

Lacy

During a mercifully brief period of my life, I spent hours every day working on a novel whose principal protagonists were a juvenile delinquent and a polar bear. That I was able to sustain any credible ambitions as a novelist, and any hopes for this particular narrative, was the direct result of Lacy's enthusiasm. That, and a sort of Decameron-like storytelling club that the two of us created.

Lacy was in her early fifties and had multiple sclerosis (MS), a progressive neurological disease that produces muscular weakness, sensory deficits, and, sometimes, emotional or personality disturbances. Her husband had died in a car accident about ten years before I met her, and Lacy didn't have children or any close family. So when her MS progressed to the point at which she needed more help than she could get from friends, neighbors, and a roster of hired nurse's aides, she sold her home in the northwest part of Philadelphia and moved to an assisted living facility downtown.

One particularly frightening feature of MS is that its progression often takes the form of a series of exacerbations and remissions, each round of which usually leaves a patient weaker and more frail. Its cyclical nature means that the devastation of MS is marked in much the same way that trenches used to mark the front lines of opposing armies. It's only by viewing the successive parallel lines as the front shifts that you can appreciate the ground that's been won or lost.

Lacy had endured three episodes over the last three years, each of which had left her temporarily wheelchair-bound. But each time, she recovered much, though not all, of her previous function. And so, when she came back to the assisted living community in late December, she had established a sort of Christmas truce with her disease. Like the peace that the Axis and Allied soldiers enjoyed near Ypres in World War I, she would enjoy a short respite before the next attack would wash over her, forcing her to give up a little more territory.

Laura, one of our most experienced hospice nurses, had been to see Lacy at her neurologist's request. Her neurologist had helped Lacy through her most recent hospitalization, which lasted almost three weeks, a stay that was complicated by a new pressure ulcer (a "bed sore" due to immobility) and a blood clot in an arm from an infected intravenous line. He knew that at some point there would be another attack, more difficult than the last, probably. He wanted Lacy to think about the option of hospice care when that happened.

Lacy knew that another relapse was likely, and perhaps even inevitable. In fact, she told Laura that she didn't want to be hospitalized again. But she also said that, no, she wouldn't want hospice.

Laura, I think, was confused by what she heard as two contradictory messages. Lacy didn't want to go back to the hospital for treatment nor did she want the care that hospice could provide in her apartment. And so Laura wondered whether Lacy understood the trajectory of MS. She asked me to stop by to see her, since Lacy's assisted living facility was only a few blocks from where we had our Wednesday hospice team meetings.

Lacy's assisted living community was in a high-rise building in the heart of the city, just off the parkway. As I rode the elevator up, looking out over the city from underneath an oddly placed sprig of leftover mistletoe, I thought about what I would say. Above all, I didn't want my visit to seem like a sales pitch. I particularly wanted to avoid the impression—reasonable under the circumstances—that Laura had asked me to try again where she had been unsuccessful.

And so when I found my way to Lacy's small one-bedroom apartment, I was prepared to be less businesslike than I would have been for a visit to any other potential patient. I decided that I would tell her I understood that she wasn't interested in thinking about hospice, now or in the future. I would say only that Laura thought that she might have other questions about hospice that I could answer.

But I needn't have worried. When Lacy answered the door, she just seemed genuinely happy to have a visitor. She smiled and ushered me in before I could deliver my prepared speech. In that first moment in the doorway I noticed she had surprisingly short grey hair and a full, almost plump face, probably the lingering result of steroid treatment during her last hospitalization. And she had crackling blue eyes that were friendly and mischievous in a ratio that was, I hoped, tilted toward the former.

Using her walker uncertainly, as if it were new to her (it was), she led me down a short hallway. In profile, silhouetted against the sun setting over the art museum at the far end of the parkway, Lacy, I noticed, was pushing the walker largely with her right hand. Her left, and her left foot, too, seemed to struggle to keep up.

The hallway led into a small living room eclectically furnished with what I imagined had been some of her favorite pieces of furniture from her house. The result was an odd mix—a sagging leather sofa, a pair of red damask upholstered armchairs, a lustrous cherry Queen Anne coffee table—that pushed aside the institutional atmosphere of her apartment. It was that mix, as much as Lacy's warm welcome and offer of tea, that made her little apartment seem like home.

Lacy gestured with her right hand toward the leather sofa, which I immediately found was enveloping and would, I thought, be very difficult to escape. I think Lacy noticed my expression because she nodded and smiled. It was her "nap couch," she said. That, and a trap for the unwary.

Sitting opposite me, with one delicate hand resting on her aluminum walker as if for moral support, Lacy seemed to be afflicted by an unusual sort of frailty. She wasn't frail in the way that, say, a ninety-year-old woman might be once illness and life events had worn her down to a core of resistance. It was more that she seemed untested, as if she hadn't been through enough to know the measure of her own strength and, therefore, was uncertain about her future.

That impression of frailty was sharpened by my realization that she was a refugee of sorts. Torn from her home not by a hurricane or tsunami, but by illness, she had landed here in an assisted living center, surrounded like a refugee by a few of her possessions. And like a refugee, she was surrounded by strangers—elderly residents, mostly—who had come to the same place twenty or thirty years later in life than she had. I guessed that her adjustment had probably not been easy.

I was surprised by how much I learned about Lacy in that first meeting. In the first five minutes of our conversation, she told me, for instance, that she'd been an adult education teacher for almost all of her professional career, after a brief stint in the Peace Corps in Namibia. And perhaps that was our first connection—we talked about the remarkable contrasts that country offered, from the escarpment along the coast, to the amazing dunes of the center, and the tiny northeast corner that had all of the country's water.

I learned, too, that she had been an avid traveler. Neither her job as a teacher, nor her husband's as a civil servant, had given them a large disposable income, but both had ensured ample vacation time. And they had used that time to travel, cheaply, throughout Africa, Asia, and South America. So naturally we talked about places we both had been. It proved to be a surprisingly large number and included many remote places. The Kalahari Desert, for instance, and Lapland, and Lake Como in northern Italy. I suppose this conversation forged a connection because these weren't the sorts of places that you'd wander into by accident, or as part of a tour.

In the course of that first rambling conversation, I was equally surprised to find that Lacy was learning quite a bit about me as well. That I was a new researcher in a new field, still a fellow in training. And that I needed to get a grant funded in the next year in order to get a faculty position at Penn. Lacy was the sort of person you could tell these things to easily, without realizing it. She had a charming curiosity that was irresistible, and she had a disarming and highly effective way of speaking in questions. Even simple statements were twisted around artfully to find a place for a question mark at the end ("We were in Soweto back in the early 80's . . . when were you there?").

Somewhere in that afternoon's conversation I forgot that my visit was supposed to be clinical, that I was supposed to determine what Lacy understood about hospice and about her illness. But there would be time for that later, I thought. As I made my way toward the door, Lacy made me promise to come back to visit. Not just a polite promise, but one that she really seemed to expect me to keep. Because her building was only a few short blocks from our team meeting office, it was quite easy for me to agree to come back the following Wednesday, if I could.

And so a week later, I retraced my steps across to her building and up to her apartment. Lacy was, if anything, stronger and more energetic. Or maybe she had been looking forward to my visit. In fact, she had laid out a plateful of digestive biscuits, which we had determined last week were our favorites for reasons which neither of us could explain. And she'd made rooibos ("redbush") tea, a somewhat astringent brew that was a staple in southern Africa. It was a taste we'd agreed we should try to acquire.

In the first few visits, every other week or so, we would talk about current events, or about the changing face of Philadelphia—

she had lived there all her life—or, as the presidential election warmed up, about politics. We spoke surprisingly little about her illness. Surprisingly, because it was on my mind and certainly on hers. And yet she would steer the conversation enthusiastically in any other direction, and I was always willing to follow her lead.

It was in the second, or maybe the third, of these visits that I happened to mention the novel I was working on at the time. It took place in a small Canadian town north of Newfoundland that is suffering from the cumulative effects of an economic recession, pervasive alcoholism, and a shrinking population. One winter the town is visited by an infestation of polar bears, which threaten to drive the rest of the human population away. Desperate, the town council solicits bids from an array of charlatans and con artists who promise to rid the town of polar bears by a variety of dubious means involving noise, electricity, offensive odors, and magnetic fields. But the council is intrigued by one proposal, from an Australian woman, who suggests turning the polar bears into a tourist attraction. The council is divided, but the majority prevails and invites the woman, and her delinquent son, to spend the upcoming winter in the town.

That's about as far as I got before Lacy started laughing—a fullthroated and surprisingly low-pitched bray that seemed to come—must have come—from someone else. She thought the idea was hilarious. She would definitely read it, she said. And she would watch the film, particularly if Julia Roberts were cast as the lead.

But then she pointed out what should have been obvious to me. That if this was the way I was spending my time, chatting with a little old lady in a nursing home and writing novels, I would never be a successful researcher. That was the only direct bit of advice that Lacy ever gave me, but she quickly softened its impact by admitting that she had the same "affliction."

She was writing a novel?

She was, and had started it when she first came to the assisted living facility. Realizing that she would have "a lot of time to think" (an understatement), and not anticipating that she would have such stimulating conversations—she nodded at me—she wanted to write a novel. She always had, in fact.

And then she told me that she had wanted to be a novelist, or at least a journalist. She had grown up in the Italian section of South Philadelphia in the early sixties. Her mother was a schoolteacher and her father worked for the city, and their house had been crammed full of books. Leather-bound classics were given pride of place in a glass case in the front room of their row house, and paperbacks were tucked everywhere else—stacked under the coffee table in the living room, mixed with cookbooks on the shelves of their harvest gold kitchen, and wedged into every available space. Her parents didn't encourage her to be a writer, at least not directly. But growing up in that house, she said, it was inevitable that she would want to.

She went to college at Penn and then spent two years in the Peace Corps, thinking that would give her "something to write about." Coming home to Philadelphia, she used her Corps stipend as a down payment on a century-old carriage house—abandoned and wisteria-strangled—in Philadelphia's Mount Airy neighborhood, only a few blocks from where I would buy an equally needy house a few years later. She got a temporary job teaching English as a second language and tried her hand at freelance writing for local papers and national magazines. She wrote short stories, topical pieces, travel essays, even editorials. Anything that might get her recognized. But her sporadic writing remained mostly uncompensated and entirely unappreciated.

So her adult education job became regularly irregular, and then permanent. She got married and restocked her life with friends. And soon she had a life that was full, with a house that needed extensive renovations, a string of adopted dogs and cats, multiple book clubs, and of course travel. And writing, once the focus of every day, receded into the background.

I knew her well enough by then to recognize her biography for the diversion that it was, designed to distract me from her novel.

But I was persistent. Much more persistent, admittedly, than I had been about talking about her illness. And eventually, I was able to coax her to talk about its story.

It was about a woman with two small boys—twins—whose husband is killed when he tries to interrupt a mugging outside a local convenience store. She feels both lonely and unsafe, and rents the garage apartment behind their house to a young single man, who would keep an eye on things and take care of the yard in exchange for cheap rent. That relationship continued for over ten years until the night of the boys' eighteenth birthday, when the man packed up his things and disappeared. The story is told from the perspective of one of her sons, now in his early fifties, who tries to fill in the rough outline of that man, and what he meant to them and to their mother, now in a nursing home.

I was intrigued—it sounded like a wonderful study of characters and, maybe, a great mystery. I wanted to hear more. Did her son find an answer? How did it end? But she wouldn't say. Maybe she was being cagey, but I suspect she just wasn't sure.

As I got up to leave, we agreed to share excerpts of what we were working on. We'd offer each other comments, and then share another excerpt. It was her suggestion, actually. She said that I would never make any progress unless I had someone looking over my shoulder. At the time, I didn't appreciate that she, too, might benefit from a reader and friendly critic.

What emerged from these exchanges, first, was that Lacy was a much better writer than I would ever be. Her physical descriptions had a vibrancy that went far beyond anything my limited gifts could produce. Succinct descriptions of a word or two would blossom into a full character as the words flew off the page, while I wrangled one reluctant adjective after another into line. And she had other gifts as well, like a knack for dialogue and a finely tuned way of describing motivations.

But it also became clear that, despite these talents, Lacy was never going to write a novel. At one meeting she gave me the same excerpt—nine or ten pages—that I'd seen before, and I realized that those ten pages were all she had. And maybe that was the limit of her gift. She could describe characters but couldn't provide the plot that she needed to get beyond that first scene in which the woman's son meets their new tenant.

So that day we skipped the usual exchange of compliments and suggestions, and talked instead about why each of us wanted to write a novel in the first place. For me it was a lark. I just wanted to see what the process of writing would be like. Borrowing her trick of turning a statement into a question, I said that I didn't really want to be a writer. But she did, didn't she?

She did, she admitted. She had thought about writing a novel almost her entire life. Not just this one, but many different ideas, at different times. She could almost divide her life into periods, defined, she said, by whatever novel she was thinking about. She hadn't made any progress on any of them.

Actually, that wasn't quite true. She had gotten into the habit of using excerpts—nine or ten pages, the same length as the piece we'd been working on—in her adult education classes as reading comprehension exercises. She was never confident that they were any good. But her students loved them, and she loved writing them.

But if she had always been "dabbling" in writing and various novel ideas, what made her want to try writing a novel in earnest now?

Her first answer was that she simply had more time now. She had given up her house and job, and lost touch with many of her friends in the neighborhood. But that didn't seem to me to be a sufficient explanation. Those life changes gave her more freedom, perhaps, but couldn't explain her motivation.

So why had she focused on writing? Why had she segregated part of every day to writing, just as she had for physical therapy? Was this an idea for a novel that she was finally happy with?

The answer that emerged was disheartening but not really unexpected. She knew that her move to assisted living in her fifties meant that, as her MS progressed, she would probably be in a nursing home in the next two or three years. And that she would probably be dead before she turned sixty. Writing a novel was one thing she had always wanted to do and, now that she had the chance, she felt that she had to try.

So writing a novel was her lifelong dream and yet she couldn't get beyond the first ten pages. I wanted to encourage her. I liked her, of course, and I wanted her to be successful. And I also loved her idea for a novel and thought that she really could write a wonderful book.

But as I sat across from Lacy that afternoon, her walker next to her chair a visible reminder of her frailty and prognosis, I was uncertain. Should I encourage her? Should I reassure her that I was sure she could finish it? (I wasn't.) That would be relatively easy. But she wouldn't believe me and, worse, she might resent my dishonesty. So I decided, instead, only to ask her whether she thought it was possible that she might not finish.

She smiled, in a sad, stiff-upper-lip way. I sensed, then, that she could appreciate that this wasn't merely a hypothetical question. If she didn't finish, and if she didn't get much further than she had, she could live with that, she said. But she had to try.

I thought then about ways I could help her. There was, for instance, a creative writing program at Penn. Maybe one of the faculty would be willing to make house calls, giving Lacy the critical guidance that she needed. But she didn't want any formal help, she said. She wanted to do this on her own. It was odd, I remember thinking, that she seemed to have forgotten her past advice to me about the value to a writer of an outside perspective.

I was quiet for a few moments, staring hard at the mug of tea—now cold—on the coffee table in front of me. I was waiting for inspiration. I let the time drag also because I wanted Lacy to see that I was thinking. I was trying to offer questions or suggestions that would be worthy.

Finally, I asked her why she was so committed to writing fiction. Before she could answer, I pointed out that she had written nonfiction pieces in the past. And I said that I remembered some of the stories about her adult education students that she had told me in the past few visits. I thought, but didn't say, that those stories had the same vibrant characters that had impressed me in the first few pages of her novel, but were all the more impressive for being cobbled on the fly out of our conversations. That was a book she could write easily, I told her.

Without waiting for her answer, I started thinking about how I could help her. I could start audiotaping our conversations, and her stories, and before long she'd have a book. But Lacy interrupted my thoughts, saying emphatically that she wanted to write a novel.

Stories of her life might interest other people, but that's not what she wanted to write. That was how her friends and neighbors and colleagues already knew her—as a teacher. A book about her teaching would simply reinforce what people thought about her. But a novel, she thought, would give people a new view of who she was, or who she could have been. And besides, God knew how many people had written books about their experiences as a teacher. That list was surely almost as long, she smiled, as the list of doctors who wrote about their patients.

Lacy talked quickly, emphatically but not angrily, and it didn't take her more than a minute to lay out her argument. I was a bit surprised—this was more personal than she had been before. But I was gratified, too, that she would share this with me—and, finally, disheartened. Because I thought there was a very good possibility that she was going to keep struggling along with a novel when another book—just as good—was so obviously within reach.

As I write this, I realize that of course I'm doing now precisely what Lacy wanted so much to avoid. Rather than a novel about juvenile delinquents and polar bears, which was beyond my own abilities, I'm writing instead about my work and my patients. And of course I'm reinforcing the image that my colleagues and friends and family have of me. But that doesn't bother me.

Why, then, did it bother Lacy so much? That was the puzzle, and the tragedy, that defined Lacy's last months. Why was she so unswerving in her commitment to writing a novel, when a nonfiction book would have been easier, and perhaps even better? It seemed like she'd rather fail as a novelist than succeed as a nonfiction writer. Of course, I knew intellectually why she had picked the course that she did. But I didn't understand it. Not really.

The Hope of Immortality

Not long after I met Lacy, I heard about a new novel whose author's story was eerily similar to hers, and which highlighted the barriers that lay in her path. In 2002, at the age of thirty-one, Stephanie Williams, a journalist, discovered that her breast cancer had rebounded vigorously despite chemotherapy and that there were no further options for a cure. Faced with the question of how she would spend the year, or perhaps two, that she had left, Stephanie chose to devote her time to the novel that she had always wanted to write.

Oddly, I already knew part of her story. I remembered reading an article she'd written in Penn's alumni magazine, when I first arrived at Penn in 1999. A hilarious account of the grim mix of smug satisfaction and envy that afflicts those of us who read alumni updates, it included her admission that these updates were, for her, a quarterly reminder of the novel that she hadn't yet written.

Through her recovery from surgery, more chemotherapy, and multiple complications and hospitalizations, Stephanie kept writing. And just as Lacy had tried to, Stephanie partnered with a friend and fellow writer for mutual encouragement. By June of 2004, she held a copy of her novel, *Enter Sandman*, privately printed. An article in *Time* after Stephanie died quoted Ellie McGrath, Stephanie's editor, as saying, "She couldn't marry the love of her life. She couldn't have a child. For a person dying so young, leaving something meaningful behind alleviated the anguish. This was her legacy."

But—and this was what helped me to understand Lacy's tenacious grip on the idea of a novel rather than nonfiction—Stephanie didn't merely want to leave something meaningful behind. She didn't just want to be remembered. Already an accomplished journalist, she was assured of that. Instead, she wanted to leave behind her a novel. That is, she wanted to be remembered in a particular way, as a writer.

Lacy, too, wanted to ensure that she would be remembered as an artist, as a writer. That is, she wanted to be remembered as someone who was creative, and she thought a novel was the best way to do this. So her novel was not just a bid for immortality, but a bid for a specific kind of immortality. The chance to live on in a particular way.

Simple Legacies

Although Lacy's goal of being remembered as a novelist seemed to me to be hopelessly out of reach, there were nevertheless countless options that would have been achievable. A nonfiction book, as I'd suggested. And many more. I've been surprised, in fact, by the legacies that my patients have been able to leave, even within the constraints of resources and time that are much more limited than Lacy's were.

One of the first hospice home visits I ever made was to an older woman with severe emphysema attributable to decades of cigarette smoking. June lived in a row house in South Philadelphia, a sort of small town in a big city where neighbors had grown up together and still took care of each other. The young girl who answered the door, I later learned, lived across the street. She was one of several neighborhood children who would stop by to check on her, to help around the house, and to run errands.

The girl led me to the living room, where June was enthroned on an overstuffed sofa that had been positioned in front of a small bay window facing the busy street. June was seated at one end and I perched at the other, but we were both half-turned toward the window—what would have been downstage—like a talk show host and her guest. That impression was reinforced whenever a neighbor would walk by, prompting June to smile, nod, and wave in what looked like an ingrained, almost royal rhythm. Clearly, she knew the neighborhood and the neighborhood knew her.

Those passersby were just a distraction, though—as I was. June's real work, and the focus of her attention, was the stacks of festive cards that were gathered in neat piles on the coffee table in front of her. June and I would talk for a few minutes—about her symptoms, or her medication regimen—and she would seem to focus on the topic. But soon her gaze would drift down to the colorful piles between us, and she'd reach for another card. She would write a few words and then slowly, laboriously, fit the card in its envelope and seal it. I noticed a stack of cards at my end of the coffee table that seemed as though they were ready for envelopes, and offered to help.

And so, as naturally as we had begun a few minutes before to talk about her shortness of breath, we talked instead about the stacks of birthday cards between us. Because that's what they were. There were well over fifty of them, all addressed to her five grandchildren. She had carefully selected cards for each of them, in themes that she thought they'd like. And she was designating each card for a future birthday that she wouldn't be there to see, writing a brief note and sending the card off into the future.

I asked June if I could read a few, and I was surprised that the notes were quite short. Most were tied loosely to anticipated events. For instance, one I remember was "Hope you're looking forward to your first Homecoming dance," intended for the September birthday of one of her granddaughters who would eventually be turning sixteen. Some offered a few words of advice, about boys or girls, about school, or about their parents.

She had got the idea, she said, from a "ladies' magazine." An article had suggested making birthday cards for yourself, a year in advance, with a note and a gift. June thought that was extraordinarily silly. Why on earth would you send yourself a birthday card and a present? But the idea made her think about her grandchildren and all of their birthdays that she would never see. And so a few days before she enrolled in hospice, June had asked one of her daughters to take her to a nearby greeting card store and had come home triumphantly with the stacks of birthday cards that now littered her coffee table. She'd give them to her children, she said, to pass them to her grandchildren on their birthdays.

I imagine one of June's granddaughters sifting through a pile of birthday cards one morning, pausing at the strangely familiar handwriting on one and slowly opening it with more restraint than she had shown so far, careful not to disrupt the looping script over the back envelope flap ("Rachel—16th"). And I imagine the close atmosphere of June's living room—the mingled smells of Pall Malls, fried food, and mothballs—somehow transmitted across the intervening years in those colored envelopes. I imagine one of her granddaughters taking all of this in—the handwriting, the short note, and maybe a lingering smell of her grandmother's house—and having her grandmother back in the room with her, if just for a moment.

But what I find most appealing about June's idea was its simplicity. It was well within her abilities, and it was elegant, too. As June showed me, there are a variety of ways to leave a legacy that will ensure that we are remembered. Legacies need not be as ambitious as a novel or a memoir. And in fact, for most of us, they probably shouldn't be. Within that range, from June's birthday cards to Stephanie Williams's novel, there is some legacy that each of my patients can leave, according to the talents they have and the time that they're given.

Life Stories

When I tried to convince Lacy to write an account of her work as a teacher, I was fishing, I suppose, for something that would capture her imagination the way that a novel apparently had. But it wasn't just a matter of pragmatism on my part. I really did believe that her stories were worth telling. Like that of the three-generation Guatemalan family in one of her classes, a teenager, her mother, and grandmother, who vied to outdo one another on the weekly vocabulary tests.

Virtually all of my patients, I think, have life stories that are worth sharing and preserving. I'm thinking in particular of the veterans that I take care of. These are men (mostly) who have survived the major wars that have defined world history over the past eighty years. I've heard enough of those stories to appreciate their value and to realize that, for every story I've heard, there are hundreds more that my patients have never, and will never, share.

They might share those stories, though, if they had an audience. The writer Joe Fiorito describes his father's gradual death from cancer in a wonderful memoir whose narrative is held together by the stories that his father tells him, including wild tales of the Mafia, monks, and bootleggers. It's not simply that he is recording his father's stories as he, the writer, sits at the bedside of his father, the storyteller. More important is that Fiorito's narrative weaves his father's history together with his own.

As his father lies weak, jaundiced, and confused, he often speaks telegraphically, in words only Fiorito could understand. ("Meow," he explains, is his father's reference to the time Fiorito's grandfather tricked one of his neighbors into eating a cat.) So Fiorito's role is more as an interpreter of their family's wild and sad history, and the storytelling becomes a collaborative effort. The net effect is that the book is almost as much Fiorito's legacy as it is his father's.

Jim Harrison uses a similar device in *Returning to Earth*, a beautiful novel about a middle-aged Chippewa man dying of ALS. The man spends much of his time and all of his remaining strength to dictate Chippewa legends and stories that were handed down to him and which, he is afraid, will be lost after his death. And so the novel is told through a final, halting dictation that weaves legend, family history, and his own story.

Although these stories from the past are intended to be legacies for the future, there may also be some immediate value in their telling. For instance, among my own patients, I've seen the sense of closure that comes with reviewing the past and making plans for a future that they won't see. This closure is particularly vivid when hospice nurses and social workers help patients to construct a life review, which is a way of collecting what are, for most of us, a series of apparently random events and accidental choices and putting them into something resembling a pattern. That pattern—of a coherent set of events, actions, thoughts, and promises—can be comforting both to patients themselves and to their families.

Watching patients go through this process can be a bit like watching a painter take a few steps back from a canvas and realize that an image has emerged from the lines and angles he has laid down. It's often not a perfect image. It may not even be the image he expected—rounder, or softer, perhaps, than what he had envisioned. And perhaps—probably, in fact—there are lines and shapes that he didn't expect. But there's something there, an essence that's recognizable. And that, often, is a good place to stop.

In addition to the sense of closure they offer to patients, these life reviews are a valuable part of hospice care because of the artifacts that they provide for family members. In fact, many of the hospice social workers I know have seen the awe with which family members, and particularly children and grandchildren, handle these histories. They've seen them displayed at memorial services and even, sometimes, brought out for reference later. When I worked as a hospice medical director, we took care of a man and then, about six months later, his wife. Our social worker and the couple's daughters used the man's life review to help his wife construct her own, and the result was two interwoven histories that could be passed on to their grandchildren.

Memorial Services

A few of my patients take the time to think carefully about the memorial service that they want. Some, perhaps, appreciate the risk of leaving their content to chance. The risk of a minister, for instance, who has never met the deceased, because he was never really much of a churchgoer. And testimonials that adhere tightly to platitudes about good works and family, carefully skirting the banalities that are better left unsaid ("He was an unexceptional man, prone to grumpiness in the morning, occasionally unkind to animals.")

In general, though, I've been struck by the paradox that most of those who take the time to plan a memorial service are those whose lives and works are already well known, even exemplary. That is, they're people whose memorial service would simply celebrate a life. But there are exceptions.

I once took care of a man with advanced prostate cancer who planned an elaborate memorial service, the size of which surprised everyone who knew him. He had been happily married to his wife for either twenty-five or twenty-seven years, depending on whom you asked. Apparently, they had been married briefly, then divorced, then remarried. This history—previously nothing more than an inside family joke—had been given new life when my patient discovered recently that he had fathered a daughter who was now about twenty-six years old. After the usual questions and recriminations subsided, though, it appeared that she was conceived during the time of their separation. At least, this was the story that the family adhered to.

This, it turned out, was his motivation for an elaborate memorial service. It was to be a chance to clarify, once and for all, his relationship with his daughter. It would be not only a memorial service, but also a public declaration of his family tree.

And just as my patient's memorial service was only partly about himself, other people have created a memorial service that is not about themselves at all but which points instead to a larger principle or belief. Peter Cicchino was a professor at the Washington College of Law in Washington, D.C., when he died in July of 2000 of colon cancer, at the age of thirty-nine. Almost exactly a month before he died, he recorded a video of an address he would have wanted to give at his memorial services. Although there are several notes that Cicchino strikes in a short video, the one I remember most comes last, an exhortation to law students to use their degrees to do good, or, as Cicchino put it, "to make the world more safe for love."

Some of my patients, though, prefer not to impose their preferences on their family. I'm thinking in particular of one man I took care of who had a large circle of friends and family and who could certainly have counted on a full house for a memorial service. But when our chaplain asked him if he'd thought about planning it, he was adamant that he didn't want to be involved at all. A memorial service, he told her, was for friends and family. It was a chance for them to arrange their memories of him however they wanted, he said, using an analogy that caught my attention. He would no more arrange his own memorial service than he would arrange his daughter's wedding. He paid for it, he said, rolling his eyes, but he left the planning to her.

Last Messages

Not all of us will have the time or the inclination to plan a memorial service, but all of us, or almost all of us, will be able to craft a few last messages for friends and family. I took care of a man once—Martin—who had many friends and just as many enemies, and just enough time before he died to distinguish carefully between the two. He did so in a way that I could identify with, by making a list. It began as eight or nine names written on the bottom of a hospital-issue cardboard box of tissues, then expanded over the space of about a week to fill half a dozen pages, front and back, of doctor's orders sheets, pinched from the nurse's station.

Next to each name he'd scrawled comments in wild, looping script: "Owes me $50"; "Wouldn't care if I wrote"; "Always looked out for Shel" (Shelley was his sister). This process took a strange, postmodern turn when he began to share the list with visitors, asking for their advice about each other. It was, in essence, his own version of a life review—a summary of those people whose friendship he was thankful for and those whose acquaintance, perhaps, he would have been better off without. Like Captain Hook in the stage version of J. M. Barrie's *Peter Pan*, who rehearses his dying words at every opportunity, Martin rehearsed his last messages on those order sheets, ensuring that they would be ready when they were needed.

Each message, taken individually, gave its recipient a unique glimpse of his or her position in Martin's life. I saw only a sample of these notes, but I got a sense of what it might be like to receive one. A few brief thoughts, an expression of gratitude, or an attempt to explain or clarify. In just a few words, Martin had managed to crystallize both a relationship and the way that he would be remembered by that person.

Together, this pile of notes helped Martin to gain some perspective on his friends and relationships, clarifying his sense of how he fit into their lives. Read carefully, and in its entirety, that stack of letters would have been a beautiful summary of his relationships, likes, dislikes, jealousies, and resentments. It was really a summary of the person that Martin was.

Ultimately, though, what was so fascinating to me about Martin's list was its gradual trend toward brevity and simplicity. It was almost as if, by putting everything on paper, he was able to whittle his relationships down to a single element. More than that, he seemed surprised, and pleased, that most of the people on his list could be summed up in a word or a phrase that was positive. In the end, our social worker was able to give Martin enough stamps and envelopes for about twenty letters, and I suspect that most of those that were mailed, finally, expressed appreciation and gratitude.

That process of writing notes was so valuable for Martin, in fact, that I've come to wonder why more of my patients don't do something similar. You could say, of course, that most of them have ample opportunity to say the sorts of things that would go into a message, and in fact many of them will. But I think that misses the point. It's not that Martin's notes expressed sentiments that he had never before shared. Perhaps that's true in some cases but, given his volubility, I'd guess only a minority. No, it's more that the act of writing, of putting pen to paper, seems to me to have an additional force in motivating closure. And maybe more significantly, just as June's birthday cards to her grandchildren did, Martin's notes provided friends and family with a tangible reminder of their relationship, and of him.

To see firsthand the impact of these sorts of notes, you only need think for a moment about other nonmedical situations in which people facing death create notes for friends and families. Across a wide range of situations—shipwrecks, mining accidents, and other natural and man-made disasters—people find time to leave a final message. Often these messages comprise just a few words scrawled on a scrap of paper or spoken into a telephone. They're created, often, in someone's final moments, under the worst possible circumstances. So it's best, perhaps, not to expect too much from them. Still, what emerges from these notes can be surprisingly beautiful.

In the Fraterville, Tennessee, mine explosion May 19, 1902, for instance, several miners were able to leave messages before their air ran out, encompassing a wide range of feelings. There were exhortations to righteousness like that of Harry Beech to his wife ("Ellen, I want you to live right and come to heaven. Raise the children the best you can.") Or like the notes of Scott Chapman ("I have found the Lord. Do change your way of living") and Powell Harmon ("Teach the children to believe in Jesus"). Other notes focus on practical advice, like the message that John Hendren left for his wife ("Bury me at Pleasant Hill if it suits you. If not bury me anywhere it suits you all. Bury me in black."). And still others offer reassurance, as in the note from Jacob Vowell ("We are not hurt but only perished for air"). The notes are on yellowed paper from a notebook that the miners would use to record weights of coal to their credit, with corners worn and dog-eared. I was surprised to see that many of them were written in exactly the same tight, upright, angular script, until I realized that this formal penmanship belonged to Jacob Vowell, who served as a scribe for others who were unable to write.

The notes of the Fraterville miners are one example in a long and tragic history of messages left by sailors, miners, and many others in dire circumstances. And so many of the themes in the Fraterville notes appear elsewhere. There can be, in fact, an eerie similarity among messages written by very different people, a hundred years apart. For instance, we can see echoes of Jacob Vowell's attempts to reassure family members in notes left by twelve miners killed in the Sago mine explosion more than a century later. "It wasn't bad," reads part of a note from mine foreman Martin Toler, Jr. "I just went to sleep."

Others have used their last opportunity to exhort family members to lead good lives, just as Harry Beech, Scott Chapman, and Powell Harmon did. Josiah Mitchell, captain of the doomed clipper ship *Hornet,* scrawled a note that reads, in part: "If I could impart advice to you, what a comfort 'twould be to me before departing hence where there is no return. . . . Put your trust in Him and make a friend of Jesus our Lord and may your lives be happy and your end peace."

Other messages include practical matters, as John Hendren's did. When Ed McNally was trapped on the ninety-seventh floor of the South Tower of the World Trade Center on September 11, he told his wife that she and their children meant the world to him. But he also divulged his secret plans to surprise her with a trip to Rome, so that she could cancel their reservations.

In thinking about these examples, and many others, my first reaction is one of regret over opportunities missed. What else might these people have written, or said, if they'd had more time—time to think, to prepare, to talk. Time to put things in perspective as Martin did. Time to pick out the right words and thoughts, and to hone them until they were perfect.

But perhaps the lack of time is a blessing of sorts. Although it's not a situation I would wish on anyone, I imagine that the pressure of the moment can have a clarifying effect. Very few of us, I think, are as rigorous about rationing our words as we could be. The pressure of time forces us to say what is most important, what truly and clearly defines the way that we'd like to be remembered.

In any case, I am amazed that so many of these messages are as heartfelt and meaningful as they are, under the circumstances. That these people, usually without warning, coaching, or time for contemplation could craft these sorts of messages is both astonishing and inspiring. And so I'm certain that people like my patients, who have months, and sometimes years, to prepare, could craft messages as well. Yet my sense is that with the exception of Martin and a few others, people dying of serious illnesses generally don't make use of these sorts of messages nearly as often as they might.

Gestures

Virtually all circumstances, it would seem, should admit the possibility of a last message—a few words on a scrap of paper or a brief telephone message. But sometimes those are out of reach. Or, sometimes, these messages can't quite capture the way in which we want to be remembered. But even then, there is the possibility of leaving legacies, of a sort.

I first recognized this possibility when I was called to see a patient just a few hours before she died. Julia had ALS and had been admitted to the ICU for treatment of a blood clot that had traveled from the veins in her leg to her lungs. That event had further weakened her already tenuous ability to breathe and required that she be placed on a ventilator.

When I met her, Julia's body had been stripped of its mass. As she lay on the bed's hard white sheets, her whitewashed face, pale grey eyes, and improbably shiny corn-silk hair were so devoid of color that she seemed ghostlike. Her slight frame barely tented the blue-and-white-striped pajamas her husband, Richard, had brought from home. The result was strangely two-dimensional, more like a coroner's chalk line drawing of where a body had been. Julia's head was immobile and tilted backward, showing skin stretched over the arch of her jaw, seemingly frozen in place as I paused at the sliding glass door of her room for five seconds, then ten. The only sign of movement was that of her frail chest in time with the ventilator.

Richard was sitting next to her faithfully, as the nurses said he had been for over twenty-four hours, gently moistening her lips with a glycerine solution. Julia's perfect opposite, Richard was a large man with an overflowing reddish-brown beard and unruly hair a few shades lighter. His bulk and the tufts of chest hair rising above the crewneck of a Temple University sweatshirt seemed to give him all the strength that Julia's illness had taken from her. Holding a thin swab in one meaty hand and a tiny paper cup in the other, he reminded me of a cartoon drawing I had seen once in an antique store in Salzburg, of a hulking bear at a tea party.

He stepped out of Julia's cubicle, closing the door carefully behind him, and slowly told me about Julia. First about her current problem and then, gradually, about the progression of her illness. About how the muscle fibers in her body had been steadily stripped away over the past nine years. And about how each setback took something from the person she had been.

He listed the elements of her identity that had been lost irrevocably along the way. Like the way she would tease an eyebrow when she was frustrated, or the way she would press her right forefinger gently on the tip of her daughters' noses to soften a rebuke. These gestures had been peeled away, slowly at first, then in bunches. Now she could no longer move or breathe on her own and was trapped, he said, in a body that was nothing more than a way station. And so early that winter morning Julia had decided she wanted to be taken off the ventilator.

Her decision wasn't unexpected. She had become increasingly frustrated, and her neurologist anticipated that Julia would eventually tire of the demands that her illness was making of her. What came as a surprise, though, was Julia's request—first to Richard and later to her sister—that she wanted to die sitting up. "Die tall" was the phrase she used in a series of coded eye blinks.

The horizontal position that she'd been forced to assume had come to define her view of the world around her and, more importantly, her place in that world. It was that position—supine, passive, vulnerable—that was the physical emblem of everything that she had lost. And so what Julia wanted most was to die sitting up. She wanted to feel that she was engaged with the world in a way that she hadn't been in the last two years—as a normal person. This was the image that she wanted her family to remember. Richard explained all this to me, pleading that we could find a way to honor her request.

In the end, her request proved to be a sort of litmus test for the ICU staff. Some of them shook their heads, declaring her request impossible. The ventilator settings would be difficult to manage, for instance, until she was disconnected. And the challenges of moving her, they said, were insurmountable.

But others—in the majority, I'm happy to say—appreciated the significance of Julia's request. They understood that Julia was "posing for eternity," to use Anatole Broyard's phrase. And so they organized, coordinated, and managed somehow to make Julia's request a reality.

Although Julia's request that afternoon surprised all of us, the idea of a final pose is not that unusual. For instance, several months after Julia died, I read about a startlingly similar gesture that Mary Lou Weisman describes in an honest and reflective book about the life and death of her son Peter. Peter lived all of his fifteen years with a particularly aggressive form of Duchenne muscular dystrophy, a disease that causes progressive weakness and eventually paralysis. Shortly before Peter died, Weisman recalls, he asked his father Larry what "impudent" means. Larry told him that it means "bold, shamelessly bold." Peter then asked his father to arrange him in an impudent position.

If Peter's last gesture defined who he was, and how he wanted to be remembered, other gestures find a broader meaning. One example that I find particularly memorable comes from a story that Eva Speter tells, in a documentary, about her evacuation from Budapest in 1944. Her train was forced to stop for "disinfection," a term that was often a euphemism for the gas chambers, and so it was with hopelessness that the passengers filed off the train to stand in front of a series of Nazi doctors. Here Speter describes what she thought were to be her last moments: "I was standing naked before the doctor and looking very proud into his eyes and [I] thought he should see . . . how a proud Jewish woman is going to die." She wanted to leave behind a legacy of sorts, but not about herself. She didn't want to be remembered as proud, per se, but rather as a representative of a proud group.

These examples all carry very different messages, of course, but they all share a sense of urgency, created by the pressures of limited time and constrained circumstances. In all of these examples, I think, there is a need to make use of every last moment in a way that conveys a message. That is a formidable challenge.

How is it possible to create a gesture—a pose—that conveys the complex meanings that Julia, Peter, and Eva wanted to impart? In thinking about this challenge, and the urgency with which it must be overcome, I'm reminded of an obscure concept from the early days of the study of developmental linguistics, or the science of how infants learn to speak. The term "holophrase" was coined by the American linguist David McNeill to describe what happens when an infant's thoughts and emotions outstrip the ability to fit words to each. The result, McNeill said, is that the infant uses a single word to express a complex meaning—what would, if uttered by an adult, require a complete sentence.

I think this analogy is illuminating because it describes—in reverse—the challenge that many of us will face in trying to make something of a very few moments. We will, some of us at least, be forced to convey complex thoughts and to encapsulate a multifaceted identity in a few moments. And we'll be forced to do so even as the ability to think and to communicate deserts us.

Inspiration versus Realism

What struck me initially about Lacy's story, and what draws all of these examples together, is the gap between the legacy that each of us would like to leave and the legacy that we're able to leave. In thinking about Lacy's dream of a novel, for instance, I'm stunned by the vast distance that separated that dream from her abilities. How did she convince herself that she could have written a novel? I wondered. How could someone who was otherwise sharp and insightful, at least about other people's self-deceptions, be so blind to her own?

If we're honest, we should acknowledge that most of us will not create anything nearly so grand as a novel. Most of us will die of chronic progressive illnesses that will overtake us gradually, slowly stripping away our ability to function, speak, and think. If this is what we can expect, is there room for grand legacies? The answer, for most of us, is no.

So we also need examples that are within reach. That is, we need examples that provide a better balance of inspiration and realism. And so for every one of us like Stephanie Williams who will use the time before we die to write a novel, there are thousands of us whose legacies must be far more limited. For some, like Lacy, a novel is out of reach but a memoir might have been possible. For others, a memorial service or a last set of messages, or birthday cards to grandchildren, are reasonable goals. And for others, a gesture like Julia's or Peter Weisman's offers the only way to be remembered.

But I need to remind myself that Lacy's novel was beyond her reach not simply because she lacked the necessary ability as a writer, but also because she obstinately refused to ask for help. Consider, for instance, that whereas Lacy steadfastly refused my offers of help and wanted to succeed, or fail, on her own, Stephanie Williams embraced those people who wanted to help her. She surely could not have completed the novel that she had envisioned without the support of a tight-knit circle of family and friends and her former editor. And near the center of this circle was Adam Fawer who, as Stephanie's writing partner, was able to help her much more effectively than I was able to help Lacy. Then, too, there was the support of the publisher and even the printer, who rearranged schedules and expedited Williams's book to ensure that it was ready before she died. The most important lesson in all of this frenetic activity, for me, is that there were so many people who were willing to help Stephanie, just as there may have been people who were willing to help Lacy.

Many of the other examples of legacies in this chapter are likewise the product of collaborations. Jacob Vowell, the Fraterville miner, was a coach and a scribe, recording last messages for the other men. Josiah Mitchell, the *Hornet*'s captain, passed paper around to the men who remained with him in the lifeboat, urging them to leave a final message. Peter Cicchino's farewell speech was a success because of the support of his colleagues and students, and became widely known when a transcript was published posthumously, again the work of his friends. And Julia's very simple final gesture was possible only because the ICU staff rose to the challenge that her last request posed for them. Lacy, too, might have been successful if she had accepted some of the support that Stephanie and others welcomed.

Lacy

My contribution to Lacy's story, if I was going to make one, seemed to hinge on the question of whether she could settle on a goal that was achievable. Achievable, that is, given her talents, resources, and time. So on the afternoon that we talked about what she could really accomplish, I wanted to know why she felt compelled to leave that legacy—her novel—that she must have known that she wouldn't finish.

The odds were certainly against her. How many novels had she started and discarded over the last twenty years? A dozen, two dozen? What made her think that this would be different?

I didn't ask her this directly, although I wanted to. Perhaps I should have, but instead, I asked her how she'd envision a book describing her teaching experiences. I knew already a book like this wasn't what she wanted to write, and I felt I knew why. Just hypothetically, though, what would it be like? What were some of the stories that she might want to tell? Was there an overarching narrative that might tie those stories together? I asked her these questions, and others, hoping that her answers, and my enthusiasm, might lead her to reconsider. I'd seen her become animated in telling stories, and I thought that I could use that enthusiasm to get her to reconsider the possibility of a book that I thought she could write.

But she wouldn't. My motives at that point were too transparent, I think. I had made a decision about what she couldn't accomplish. And my decision wasn't one she wanted to hear.

I realized then that I had broken one of the rules of our relationship. She was happy, it seemed, to "work" with me on a novel that she knew she would never finish. Just as I would work with her on mine. But I had disrupted this equilibrium when I said that her goal wasn't realistic. Much worse, I had unknowingly tricked her into breaking the rules by admitting this to herself.

Perhaps my mistake was for the best, because I think I would have found it very difficult to maintain a relationship like that. I was perfectly happy to use my own novel as window dressing as long as I was helping Lacy. Indeed, after our first few conversations it had become obvious to me at least that my novel didn't have much of a future. What did I know about polar bears, after all? Still, I felt the time I was spending with Lacy was justified by whatever help and encouragement I was offering. Take that away though, and our time together, ostensibly "working," was a farce.

Our relationship didn't end that afternoon. For another three months, I continued to visit Lacy's building every few weeks, since our hospice had several patients there. I'd stop in to see her, less often, certainly, but still regularly. Sometimes she would say she was too tired for company. She'd blame her medications, or a sleepless night. But when she felt well enough, we would continue to share notes about writing and writers, including recommendations of books we had read. We felt more free, or at least I did, to talk about other things. It was, oddly, a more comfortable relationship, much closer to that first conversation we had a few months earlier.

Closer to that first conversation, but not quite the same. I may have forgotten about my own novel, but I remembered Lacy's. And I remembered the possibility of a nonfiction book. I don't recall that we ever talked about either again, although we may have in passing. Still, I wondered—as I still do—whether I gave up too easily. Could Lacy have written her novel? Could her story have had the ending that, say, Stephanie Williams's story did?

As I think about it now, I wonder whether perhaps Lacy didn't really want to finish that novel at all. Certainly, she had been toying with the idea for years. It seems possible that she had given up any expectation of finishing and instead just needed to feel that she had made a legitimate attempt. That's an attractive answer to me, because it absolves me of responsibility. It says, in effect, that there's nothing more I could have done to help. Even better, perhaps, it suggests that I was more helpful than I knew. My well-meaning encouragement to consider nonfiction instead might have been just what Lacy needed to lay that novel to rest.

But I can't make myself believe this, much as I'd like to. There are far too many people like Peter Cicchino and Stephanie Williams who were able to create the legacies that they wanted to, once they had the help that they needed. So the idea that I did all I could offers a hollow sort of reassurance. Besides, I discovered later that Lacy's time was not nearly as limited as we'd thought. Although I lost touch with her after she moved to another apartment, much later I happened to meet her neurologist. He told me that Lacy's MS had become quiescent after the prolonged hospital stay that brought her to the assisted living facility, and that the truce she had enjoyed when I met her had held. In fact, he said, she had remained in reasonably good health for the next five years until she was diagnosed with metastatic colon cancer and died a few months later. So she had five years of good health and what was, clearly, a tenacious resolve to write. Could she have finished a novel in the time that she had? She couldn't have done it on her own nor, almost certainly, with whatever meager advice I was able to provide. But perhaps with enough support and encouragement, she could have left the legacy that she imagined.

EIGHT

Ladislaw

Giving and Helping

Ladislaw

Ladislaw was quick to dismiss much of the world as "silly." Like my recommendation that he take a long-acting pain medication, for instance. "Why? That's silly. What I'm taking works perfectly well." The fact that he had to wake up two or three times every night to take a dose didn't dissuade him. "If that's when I need my medication, then that's when I will take it."

Even his oncologist encountered Ladislaw's derision when he recommended a chemotherapy drug in the form of a pill to be taken once a day. "A pill? That's like asking a mechanic to fix an engine and then handing him a screwdriver. How will a pill treat cancer?"

Nor was he mollified by the oncologist's argument that although the pill was not terribly effective, at least it didn't have any significant side effects. "I should take this pill because it doesn't make me sick? What sort of logic is that?" Even his oncologist had to admit that Ladislaw had a point.

And the cancer that would kill him, an adenocarcinoma of unknown origin, received his particular scorn. He couldn't understand—and certainly couldn't respect—a cancer that steadfastly resisted efforts to categorize it, and one which behaved so erratically. The cancer appeared in his lungs, for instance, although he had no history of smoking. And it seemed to regress spontaneously at first, only to grow while he was receiving chemotherapy. It was, he thought, a silly disease to die from.

In short, Ladislaw was motivated—driven—by reason and logic. And he was disturbed in an almost visceral way when the world failed to operate in the rational, regimented way that he expected it to. But if he was disturbed by people and events that were not purely rational, I'm sure he was no longer surprised.

In the early days of World War II, Ladislaw had escaped from Warsaw, where he had been an engineering student. On the day that Germany invaded Poland, he saw, more clearly than most, I think, what the future held for all Poles—Jews and non-Jews alike. So he threw his most prized possessions into a trunk and made his way slowly westward through Sweden, to Norway, and ultimately to the United States. He had just gotten settled in Philadelphia working for an engineering company when he was drafted into the Army and sent back to Europe.

He wasn't resentful about that twist of fate, though he certainly could have been. What annoyed him most, characteristically, was the fact that the Army handed him—a trained engineer—a rifle. It was the one piece of machinery that he wasn't at all familiar with. He hated to think of the other side of that error, he told me once. Did the same Army take a boy out of high school, hand him a slide rule, and tell him to build a bridge?

Ladislaw survived the war without injury and also, as he tells it, without doing much of anything. The Army eventually recognized his talents, in a way, and he spent the remaining months of the war doing maintenance work at several camps well away from active fighting. He emerged somewhat relieved, but more puzzled, that his participation hadn't influenced the course of events even a bit. That's not quite true, actually. He did say that he had made some improvements to the kitchen equipment in several camps. The one which he was most proud of was a mechanism to filter grease in the kitchen fryer. It was, as he described it, a modest victory of order and efficiency over chaos.

I learned all of this gradually, over the course of perhaps a half-dozen visits to our palliative-care clinic at the Philadelphia VA hospital. I had just finished my fellowship, and I worked part-time at the VA with several wonderful people—Lucy Pierre, Jack Coffey, and Priscilla Kissick—who were dedicated to providing good care to patients near the end of life. Together, we decided to create an outpatient palliative care clinic, which was a novelty at the time. Previously, most efforts in the United States to improve end-of-life care had either provided hospice care in patients' homes or offered palliative-care consults in hospitals. In our clinic we focused on patients who were still living at home, and who were not yet sick enough to be hospitalized, or to enroll in hospice. Over the three years that we ran the clinic, we helped patients and families to make decisions about treatment, we orchestrated hospice referrals, and we helped with management of pain and other symptoms.

But Ladislaw wasn't referred to us for any of these reasons. Instead, he came to get our advice about whether he should enroll in one of several studies of experimental cancer therapies that were going on at the University of Pennsylvania. His oncologist had told me that Ladislaw wanted to enroll in a study, but that Ladislaw's daughter, who has been his main source of support since his wife had died a few years earlier, was vehemently opposed. His oncologist seemed to side with Ladislaw's daughter. Ladislaw was too sick, he said, and probably wouldn't even be eligible for a trial.

The oncologist also told me a little about Ladislaw, just enough to make me wonder why he was so determined to enroll in a Phase I trial. For instance, Ladislaw was "very organized," the kind of patient who takes notes at clinic visits, keeps a folder of his medical paperwork, and questions everything. Not the sort of person, I thought, who would chase after a slim hope of benefit offered by an experimental treatment.

I first met Ladislaw in our clinic the week after his oncologist had called me. Slender to the point of being gaunt, with wavy white hair and expansive flapping limbs, he had tangled eyebrows cantilevered out over a rough-hewn face. He looked as if he'd been carved—imprecisely, with an exceptionally blunt chisel—from a block of old-growth hickory. And that arboreal impression was heightened by his clothes, a complex brown Harris Tweed suit and a sweater of indeterminate green.

But he also had a restless energy that was astonishing, given how advanced his cancer had become. When I called his name in the waiting room, he popped upright and marched enthusiastically down the hall in front of me, stepping unprompted into the only open room. I followed, closing the door behind me, and dropped into one of the remaining seats.

As we sized each other up, there was a perfunctory knock on the door, which opened to reveal an attractive fortyish blond woman. She was impeccably dressed in a charcoal suit, carried a Louis Vuitton handbag, and was wearing considerably more makeup than was strictly necessary for a visit to a VA hospital. As she stood over us, her pointed stare shifting like a searchlight back and forth between Ladislaw and me, I recognized the woman who had been sitting next to him in the waiting room.

"You have met me," he said, shrugging angular shoulders, "and now you have met my daughter Emma." He smiled—apologetically to me and a bit defiantly at his daughter. "So now we can begin."

I introduced myself and apologized. But Emma was less upset with me for closing the door on her than she was with her father for making what seemed, in retrospect, like a desperate bid for freedom. In fact, that was more or less the way she seemed to treat her father, as a good-natured but not particularly well-behaved puppy who would get into all sorts of mischief if he weren't kept on a tight leash.

I began the visit as I usually do, by asking Ladislaw to tell me what he knew about his cancer and his prognosis. But with Emma sitting between us, blocking questions and generally interfering, Ladislaw's answers always seemed to be eclipsed by his daughter's. With what seemed like resignation, he would usually pause to let Emma go first. But as I got to know Ladislaw better, that resignation began to seem more like patience, as if he were a professor giving a student a chance to convince him that, maybe, this time, she would provide the correct response.

Slowly, through this triangle of questions and answers, it became clear that he—they—knew that Ladislaw had widely metastatic cancer. They knew, too, that this diagnosis conferred a very poor prognosis. In fact, since his cancer was first diagnosed eight months before, it had proved unstoppable. Ladislaw had been through several rounds of chemotherapy without any success. He and Emma had both seen all too clearly its side effects, including severe nausea and fatigue. And so they both understood that Ladislaw's treatment options were very limited.

This was when Ladislaw told me about his oncologist's offer to give him chemotherapy in the form of a pill, and about the oncologist's grudging admission that it wouldn't really be effective. This, for Ladislaw, was the final piece of evidence, as if one were needed, that there were no treatment options left. "Other than that pill," he waved a hand dismissively, "there is nothing else he can do. So I want to learn about experiments that are open."

And what did he know about these "experiments"?

Ladislaw answered quickly, for the first time, preempting any answer from his daughter. They were, he said, experiments to test the safety of new drugs. This was true. In fact, the trials that his oncologist had mentioned to me were all Phase I trials, which are the first tests of new drugs in humans. Ladislaw also knew that the main goal of such trials was to determine the maximum dose that patients could tolerate.

When I said I was impressed by how well he understood the design of these trials, my compliment received the same wave with which he had dismissed the oncologist's "pill." It was common sense, he said. And besides, this method of testing was exactly the same method that "anyone" (meaning, I suppose anyone who was an engineer), would use to evaluate the structural integrity of building materials. "Testing to destruction," he called it. A procedure of stressing a structure until it failed, in order to determine how much stress it could withstand. Although I found this analogy a bit gruesome, and while I suspected that my colleagues who ran Phase I trials wouldn't appreciate it either, I had to admit that it was apt.

So he understood that the goal of these trials was to test safety, and that there was no real chance of a meaningful benefit? Before he could answer, though, Emma interrupted him.

"No benefit. See? That means it won't help you. At all. Not even a little bit." She punctuated each point with jabs of a forefinger on the small table that separated the two of them, each one a few inches closer to her father, like the footsteps of an advancing army of logic.

But Ladislaw was unperturbed. Like a long-suffering professor, he knew from hard-won experience that all classroom chaos eventually subsides. And besides, I think we both recognized that Emma's arguments were irrelevant. Ladislaw understood as well as I did that these were, truly, "experiments" that wouldn't help him.

So why, then, did he want to enroll in one?

Up until then, he had been willing to speak, and even eager to do so, when he had the opportunity. But now he was strangely reticent. He would say only that he wanted to be "useful."

And then I understood his reluctance. That answer, which seemed to me to be harmless enough, unleashed a barrage from Emma. She chastised him, first, for talking about enrolling in experiments of "new chemicals" that wouldn't help, "even according to this doctor." And she gave me the same—apparently inherited—wave that her father used so disparagingly. "And it's one thing to talk about no benefits, but what about the side effects?"

Now, I realized, she was talking to me. How much was her father going to have to suffer, she asked? It was just irresponsible, what he was going to do.

At this point in the conversation I wasn't sure whether she was referring to her father or, as I began to suspect, to me. At the very least, she said, Ladislaw shouldn't do this without consulting his other daughter.

I must have looked alarmed—Emma at this dose was unpleasant, and at twice the dose would probably be toxic—because Ladislaw smiled and laid a hubcap-sized hand on my arm.

"Don't worry, she is in California. But," he gave my forearm a warning squeeze, "she is a nurse."

Ladislaw wouldn't say anything more. He just smiled, shrugging his thin shoulders in a way that had already become a signal to me to let things be. And so I suggested that I would see if there were any trials open at Penn that he would be eligible for.

That seemed to please Ladislaw more than Emma, but they were both satisfied enough that we could move on to other topics. Ladislaw's living situation, for instance, and the help he was going to need as he got weaker. And the abdominal pain that I was worried might be due to liver metastases.

As they left an hour later, though, I realized that the reason he was referred in the first place—"advice" about a Phase I trial—was no closer to a resolution than it had been that morning. Still, I didn't feel like I had failed. Ladislaw clearly had his reasons for wanting to participate in a trial. And just as clearly he wasn't willing to say any more in front of his daughter, for which I could hardly blame him. So as I walked out to the waiting room to fetch my next patient, reminding myself not to leave a wife or daughter behind, I decided that at his next visit I would try to talk to Ladislaw alone.

Acts of Altruism

It took me more than two weeks to search for available trials, and so I had ample time to think about Ladislaw's motivations for participating in one. Yet I could make little headway. What confused me most was Ladislaw's claim that he wanted to be "useful."

I found this motivation particularly difficult to understand because I had trouble reconciling it with what I saw—perhaps incorrectly—as Ladislaw's pragmatic, workmanlike attitude toward life. As far as I could tell, Ladislaw had always been careful and rational. In particular, his approach to his treatment had been nothing if not logical. He'd carefully weighed the risks and potential benefits of his options and he'd quickly rejected those treatments, like the scorned chemotherapy "pill," that did not make sense to him.

My error, I think, was that I mistook Ladislaw's careful balancing of risks and potential benefits—his endless questions to the oncologists, and his notepad record of every suggestion—for crotchety self-interest. And so I had trouble imagining that Ladislaw might suddenly have become altruistic. That I came to this conclusion was largely the result of the examples of altruism near the end of life that I had seen before I met Ladislaw.

In my own mind, the most vibrant example of such altruism was the story of Father Damien. I grew up in Hawaii, where Father Damien's story was related to schoolchildren with the same religious reverence that I imagine was devoted in mainland schools to the life of George Washington. So we all learned about how Father Damien spent his last years dying of leprosy in the leper colony on the island of Molokai. He was, we were taught, a persistent letter writer and gadfly to the regional authorities. He was also a tireless worker and organizer, cleaning, organizing, acting in turns as a civil engineer, a sanitation worker, a teacher, a mayor, and of course a priest. "There is so much left to do" was his constant response to those who advised him to slow down and to conserve his energy.

It was this dogged persistence in helping others even in the last weeks of his life that contributed to the mix of spiritual awe and hometown pride with which Father Damien was, and is, regarded in Hawaii. There is a statue outside the state capitol in his honor, for instance, and a state holiday (April 15) in his name. And for Catholics, at least, there is a feast day to honor his beatification. Father Damien is a perfect example of someone who used his last months of life to help others.

A perfect example, but one that really only illustrates the way that he had lived his life. Because we also learned that when Father Damien, born Jozef de Veuster, arrived in 1863, the colony was little more than a concentration camp. Damien lived among the lepers for sixteen years, transforming the colony into a sort of sanctuary where those afflicted by leprosy, although they continued to be confined involuntarily, could find something resembling peace and comfort. We learned, too, about how he shared his home and his possessions until finally, as everyone expected, he began to show evidence of the disease. Aware that his diagnosis was not merely a threat to him, but to all that he had accomplished, he devoted his final year to securing the future of all that he had built.

So when I thought of altruism in the last months of life, it was examples like Father Damien's that came most readily to mind. And I couldn't see how Ladislaw's story fit this mold. When I looked past his daughter at Ladislaw as he sat in our clinic, I thought I saw someone whose past choices were objective and calculating. Not always self-interested, perhaps, but certainly not prone to wildly uplifting flights of spirituality and a sense of connection with others that might drive an altruistic bid to participate in risky research.

Instead, what I saw in Ladislaw's plan to be "useful," or at least what I thought I saw, was the choice of someone who had been transformed by his illness. Ladislaw, it seemed, had accepted the imminence of his death and had, somehow, rearranged his priorities. And that, more than anything, was what puzzled me. Not that Ladislaw or anyone else might behave altruistically. There are surely enough examples around us every day to make this entirely plausible. Instead, what I thought I saw that day in clinic was a fundamental rearrangement of his priorities, an acute onset of altruism, prompted by his illness and approaching death.

But I wasn't sure that I believed what I saw. Could a terminal diagnosis really make someone like Ladislaw into an altruist? Could a terminal diagnosis rearrange his priorities so substantially as to make the needs of others more important than his own?

Becoming Altruistic

That I was skeptical about such a transformation in Ladislaw's case is probably attributable more to a dour view of human nature than to any evidence or personal experience. This was not something I had given any thought to, and thus had not paid any attention to in my own patients. But current events conspired to rearrange my own thinking about Ladislaw and his desire to be useful.

It was on one of my clinic days, in fact—a Tuesday—shortly after I first met Ladislaw, that the other physicians and I found ourselves gathered around a computer in a colleague's office, watching the events of September 11 unfold in a series of slowly loading images. And I noticed, probably more than I otherwise would have, how many stories of altruism emerged from those accounts. The most visible, perhaps, was that of United Flight 93, whose passengers succeeded in crashing the plane to prevent it from reaching its target in Washington, D.C. But there were hundreds of other examples, too, that filtered out in the weeks and months that followed.

These examples didn't change my view of Ladislaw, at least not immediately. They were too far apart, really, and came from a wholly different world. Still, the stories from that day prompted me to think about altruism in Ladislaw's case, and elsewhere. And there are, in fact, a wide variety of ways in which altruism appears near the end of life in those with serious illness. A few of my patients, for instance, have financial resources and focus on using that money to do good. Others don't have money but do have talent and experience to share. Others, perhaps, have energy to rally and organize. And for some of us, the best opportunity to help others lies in the illness that afflicts us, and the possibility of participation in research.

Giving

Some of us, faced with the possibility of death and motivated by the desire to help others, will have extensive resources that we can deploy. Not many of us, certainly, but a few. These are the examples of altruism that are highly visible.

For the most part, I've worked in overcrowded university hospitals, state institutions, and in the VA health care system. These are not settings, generally, that bring me into contact with wealthy patients. However, there have been a few exceptions.

The patient I remember best was a phenomenally successful businessman, well known to the staff at the hospital where I worked. His advanced age—he was in his eighties—had brought a growing list of medical problems that had given him increasing familiarity with the hospital over the past few years. Never much of a philanthropist, the story went, he had recently become wildly generous to the hospital and its affiliated university. He supported several endowed chairs for faculty, scholarships for students, and even an entire hospital wing shortly before he died.

I remember this story so clearly because, at least in the version that I heard, it was the proximity of death that motivated this man's altruism. Left, I suppose, with more money than his children could possibly need, he turned to philanthropy. And in doing so, he did a great deal of good.

But I also remember his story because of the diverse ways in which his gifts were perceived. There were those, of course, who saw them as evidence of pure altruism. The hospital administration was in this camp, as were many of the physicians who took care of him. This was a man, they said, who wanted to use his substantial resources to help people.

But there were others whose views were more nuanced. Several of the nurses in the cardiac ICU who knew him, for instance, thought that he was motivated not so much by pure altruism as by a desire to be remembered. He didn't merely want to be generous, they said, he wanted to be remembered as generous. Others were forthrightly cynical, suggesting that these gifts were little more than an insurance policy, guaranteeing him the best possible care.

These conversations weren't hidden. In fact, his increasingly frequent hospitalizations and almost ceremonial clinic visits reliably prompted these sorts of discussions. And so, as a result, what I remember most clearly is not the good that this man did for the hospital and its university, but rather the second-guessing that surrounded his motives.

In stark contrast, I can think of a man with Parkinson's disease I took care of once. Far from wealthy, he and his wife lived in a small row house in South Philadelphia. That home was virtually all they owned. I knew this because one of their concerns was that they would lose even the house—the only asset they could leave to their children—to pay their medical bills.

Given this history, I was surprised when the man announced shyly at one clinic visit that he had brought me a present. Without waiting for me to respond and, I think, anticipating an awkward refusal, he reached into a plastic shopping bag and gingerly removed a small pen case. He opened it, passing it to me gently across the table, the tremor in his hands subsiding as he did so. I knew that Parkinson's typically causes a resting tremor that disappears with movement. But it was difficult not to infer a symbolic meaning as I saw his hand become relaxed, and confident, in that gesture.

The gift, it turned out, was a well-used mechanical pen and pencil set. Scratched and scuffed with use, the two were resting uncomfortably in an equally well-used plastic case that, on close inspection, seemed to have been made for another set entirely. The pen and pencil matched each other, though, as my patient was quick to point out.

The VA has rather strict rules about accepting gifts from patients, and I have my own self-imposed rule that can be reduced, more or less, to "nothing of more than sentimental value." This gift seemed to fit, and besides, my patient's shyness and awkwardness made me nervous that he would be offended by a refusal, even a refusal on ethical grounds.

So I thanked him and then paused, unsure whether to ask him why on earth he was giving me a well-used pen and pencil set. He seemed reluctant to say more and so his wife volunteered a partial explanation. Her husband, she explained, collected old pens and pencils. He would pick them up at flea markets and garage sales. After cleaning them and finding a case that fit, more or less, he would sell them for a bit more at yard sales in the neighborhood, making a few cents on each exchange.

Then my patient awkwardly picked up the story. He was grateful for all of the care he had received from the VA over the years, he said, and he wanted to give something back. But he had nothing, really, to give. Nothing except a stock of pens that he hadn't yet resold. And so he had spent the last few weeks sorting through what surely must have been a large pile, finding the best specimens, and cases that were at least close to the originals.

I learned later that he had given similar gifts to many others who had taken care of him. He did not distinguish much among us. I noted just a bit proudly that whereas I received both a pen and pencil, one of my colleagues, who had known our patient for much longer, had received only a pen. Proudly, that is, until my colleague pointed out that at least his pen worked. He was right. Neither of my writing implements was functional. Still, I put them in a repurposed coffee mug on my desk and, over the years, they've gained the dignity of a sort of weathered aristocracy among my motley collection of battered pencils and disposable pens.

Teaching

Not all of my patients have a large pen collection and even fewer, unfortunately, can afford to endow a professorship. But there are a variety of other forms that altruism takes near the end of life. As a medical student, I took care of a patient who had the misfortune of having a strange neurodegenerative disorder that no one could diagnose. Nina's condition was characterized by progressive weakness, sensory loss and intermittent pain. Worse, her complaints of pain initially led several of her doctors to conclude that she was inventing her symptoms in order to obtain pain medications. But it eventually became obvious that her disease was all too real, although that acknowledgment, and countless examinations, tests, scans, and biopsies, were unable to assign a cause or suggest a treatment.

Nina was admitted to our neurology service not for a diagnostic workup—her doctors had long since lost hope of putting a name to her illness—but for symptomatic treatment of the muscle spasms that were causing her considerable discomfort. I was assigned to take care of her and was surprised to find, when I met her, that she had kept detailed records of virtually every aspect of her care. In fact, she had with her a black-and-white speckled composition notebook, with a small red 4 on the upper right-hand corner of the front cover, which was organized into columns labeled "Symptoms," "Date," "Treatment," and "Outcome."

This was a treasure trove of data for a busy medical student who was faced with the daunting task of learning everything there is to know about a patient with a complex history in time to present a coherent summary the following morning. But Nina wouldn't let me take the notebook with me, not even to make a copy. So I sat by her bedside for hours that night, reading through it, taking notes, and asking questions.

Thanks largely to her notebook, the next morning I was able to give an award-winning summary of her symptoms. And I was prepared for all of the questions that the neurologist asked me. When the muscle spasms had started, for instance, and how they had progressed, and what made them better or worse. All of his questions, that is, except for one.

As we were concluding our discussion in the conference room, the neurologist asked me why Nina had been keeping her diary all these years. I had no idea, since I hadn't thought to ask. So I guessed. It was, perhaps, a favor that she did for medical students?

The neurologist smiled. He had a famously odd sense of humor, as well as a high tolerance for slow-witted medical students. He also knew Nina well and had taken care of her on multiple previous admissions. He knew that her notebooks weren't intended as a training aid for students. At least, not exactly.

He explained to the group what I should have been able to tell them. Nina had become frustrated by medicine's failure to find a diagnosis. Her frustration led her to avoid doctors entirely for a time, trying a variety of complementary medical therapies. Finally, she channeled her frustration and began keeping a diary.

Her diary, he explained, was essentially a case report. Influenced, perhaps, by all of the poking and prodding and studying that she had had to endure, she began thinking of herself as an experiment of sorts. An oddity that others could learn from. And so she began keeping her notebook. Only a rough diary at first, it eventually became a meticulous record of everything about her disease. The neurologist said that Nina hoped that these records might someday help to identify whatever disease she had so that others in the future might benefit from her experience.

Although her dedication was unique, she is hardly the only person who used a terminal illness as an opportunity to learn and to teach. Peruse the bookshelves of your local bookstore and you'll find an astoundingly long row of illness memoirs. It seems that there is something close to a compulsion to record our illnesses and the experiences they bring. These memoirs—many of them at least—seem to be driven by a desire to teach, to share.

There are many more examples, of course, each a unique view of, and from, a terminal illness. In fact, it's interesting to me how my view of a particular illness can be defined, or at least framed, by a particularly vivid account. Harold Brodkey's beautifully chiseled account of his battle with AIDS, for instance. Or Anatole Broyard's lyrical account of his last year of life as he was dying of prostate cancer. Or Tim McLaurin's rough and tumultuous account of his battle with multiple myeloma, whose roller coaster of indignities is mirrored perfectly in the shifting tone of his book.

There have been journalists like Natalie Spingarn, Max Lerner and Stewart Alsop, whose accounts read like dispatches from the front lines of their battles, and which were intended at least in part to inform and educate the public. And scientists like Stephen Jay Gould whose essay on the dangers of misinterpreting prognostic estimates is perhaps the single most widely cited article in online cancer discussion groups. And of course there have been teachers like Randy Pausch whose "Last Lecture" drew international attention. And there are others such as Peter Cicchino and Archie Hanlan whose final days were spent crafting lessons. Hanlan in particular was annoyed, he says, by those who found his articles and lectures to be a "moving experience." His goal, he chides them, was not to "move" people, or to inspire them. Instead, he wanted to teach.

But my favorite example comes not from a novelist or journalist. Roger Bone was widely regarded as the father of modern intensive care medicine. A researcher, clinician, and teacher, he has arguably done more than anyone else to advance the field of critical care. And so it was surprising and perhaps more than a little ironic when his diagnosis of advanced renal cancer prompted him to become an aggressive advocate for palliative care. He used the standing that he had gained in academic medicine to write, and to speak to physicians and other health care providers.

All of these people were teachers who watched, and listened, and passed on what they'd learned to others who might, perhaps, face the same experiences someday. This self-appointed role reminds me of a tradition among recreational cyclists that the first rider in a group should be alert for potholes, sewer grates, or other obstacles that are likely to pose a threat to bicycles traveling very fast on very skinny wheels. That person then points out those obstacles to riders who are following behind. Doing so is an obligation, certainly, and often an obligation that is enforced through norms in a riding group. But it's an obligation that brings with it a sense of purpose, and even reward, as obstacles are identified and, one hopes, avoided, as the long train of riders picks up the signal, passing it back down the line. This is how I see people like Gould and Spingarn and Hanlan and Broyard and even my patient, with her diary. Riding at the front of the pack, they were all watching with a ready alertness and sharing what they saw with those who would come later.

Doing

If some people give, and some teach, there are others who simply do. The best example of this I've ever seen, by a wide margin, is Alex Scott, a girl who used to live only a few blocks away from me in the Philadelphia suburbs. When she was only one year old, Alex was diagnosed with neuroblastoma, a particularly resistant childhood cancer that is often fatal, and which can cause devastating neurological complications. When she was four years old, she underwent a stem-cell transplant, paired with intensive chemotherapy, in hopes of slowing her cancer's progression. It was during that hospitalization that she first had the idea of organizing an annual lemonade stand to raise money for pediatric cancer research.

The first stand raised a modest amount, as did the second. But the third generated considerable local news coverage and gave the project an energy that astonished Alex's parents. No longer just a pet project within the family, Alex's idea had become a public phenomenon. In 2002 her parents established a fund in her name that brought in $40,000 by the end of the year. National attention continued to grow until, in 2004, Alex's Lemonade Stand had become a nationwide event, with stands in every state. By the time that Alex died that August, she had raised over $1 million for pediatric cancer research. A year after her death Alex's Lemonade Stand became a registered public charity that continues to raise millions of dollars every year.

I heard about the later phases of Alex's story as it unfolded. She was, for a time, something of a media celebrity in Philadelphia and certainly at the Children's Hospital of Philadelphia (CHOP), where she received much of her care. What I heard was inspirational. But while I was entirely willing to be inspired, I had questions, too.

How did a grand idea like this come to a four-year old? How did her parents react? Were they skeptical? Supportive? Protective? And how did such an enormous project change the way that Alex spent the last years of her life? Did it take time away from other things that she could have done? There were no answers to questions like these in the uniformly energetic and inspirational press releases that chronicled her successes. So I asked her parents, Jay and Liz Scott, to help me understand how this path of altruism unfolded for Alex, and what it meant for her, and for all of them.

They tried to explain, first, where the idea of raising money for pediatric cancer came from. "Tried," because they weren't quite sure. Alex had been seen by specialists in several cities, they said, and had been told, finally, that nothing more could be done. The best they could do, Alex's doctors said, was to make Alex comfortable and to give her a chance to enjoy whatever time she had left.

But her parents heard of an experimental treatment at CHOP and traveled to Philadelphia. That treatment proved so effective, at least in the short term, that she was eligible for a stem cell transplant, which she received a short time later. And it was this double step from hopelessness—through research—to a potentially effective transplant, her parents thought, that planted the idea in Alex's mind that medical research offered promise.

In addition, though, they thought Alex was unusually perceptive. Jay told me that as she went through treatment she'd met—and said goodbye to—dozens of children. Some of them had been cured, but many others had died. And in all of those interactions, Jay said, Alex had paid attention. She saw that the children around her were unhappy, and she wanted to do something to help.

Yet when Alex first raised the idea of setting up a lemonade stand, Jay and Liz misunderstood. They thought that Alex wanted to earn money for herself. So Liz said that they didn't try to dissuade her, although they weren't entirely supportive, either. But over the course of that winter Alex made it clear that she didn't want the money for herself, but rather for research for pediatric cancer.

At first Jay and Liz were amused. Liz admitted that she thought Alex's idea was "sweet" and "kind of funny." Well-meaning, and certainly admirable, but overly ambitious. How could $5 or $10 make a meaningful contribution to cancer research?

But Alex was persistent, and Jay and Liz were forced to examine their own reactions to Alex's plan and to understand their reluctance. In part, they said, they were afraid that Alex would be disappointed. It seemed very likely that Alex's fundraising wouldn't meet her goals. And it was possible that her declining health might be a barrier. So they searched for a fine balance between protecting Alex on one hand, and letting her do what she felt she had to do on the other.

For instance, when they moved from Connecticut to Philadelphia, Jay and Liz knew that it would be harder for Alex to raise money without their old circle of friends and neighbors. They worried that her second stand would not produce the $2,000 that her first stand had. But instead of persuading Alex to give up, they suggested postponing the stand until they had been in Philadelphia longer. By that fall, they said, Alex would know more people and would have the support of her school. Even with that postponement, Alex's stand that year raised only $700. But Alex was philosophical. She suggested to her parents that perhaps a cold, rainy fall day was not the best time to have a lemonade stand and that next year they should go back to Alex's original plan and set it up in the summer as she had wanted initially. They did, and raised $12,000.

Any way I looked at it, Alex's seemed like a remarkable success story. Even more so as her project drew local and then national media attention. National news coverage, for instance, and an appearance on *Oprah*.

But I wondered whether this project, and its success, had a cost. Were there "normal kid things" that Alex couldn't do because she was spending time on her lemonade stands? Were there disadvantages spending this amount of time and energy on raising money to help others?

Jay and Liz were quick to clarify, first, that Alex's project didn't really gain a national presence until the last six months or so of her life. That explosion was coincident with Alex's bold—and apparently spontaneous—boast to a reporter that she would raise $1 million. So the actual portion of her life that Alex devoted to altruism was less than what the national news coverage, for instance, might have portrayed.

But were there disadvantages to the time that she did spend? I'm sure that Jay and Liz thought I was fixated on this, but I couldn't shake the idea that Alex was giving up the life of a more normal kid to do this. Giving up sleepovers, for instance, and evenings talking with friends.

Jay and Liz were emphatic. They didn't think Alex had any regrets for the way that she had spent her time. Nor did they regret the support that they gave her.

And I realized, then, that I had been looking at Alex's life in the wrong way entirely. It wasn't as if she had given up some things in order to follow her dream of raising $1 million for pediatric cancer research. She wasn't choosing altruism instead of other things at all. It was more, Jay said, as if she did it all. It was as if she had packed eighty years of living into eight.

More important, perhaps, her lemonade stands and the publicity they generated often gave Alex opportunities and experiences that most "normal" kids would love to have. For instance, a large international company sponsored a trip for her family to Disney World, which proved to be the last trip their family would take. Her celebrity led, too, to shopping trips to New York and Chicago with friends and family. (Jay still remembers the credit card bill from those trips). And prime seats, with friends, at a concert with a chance for them all to meet the performers. These were all opportunities and experiences that Alex could share with friends and family, and which would have been out of reach for most children.

But Jay and Liz pointed out some other costs that I hadn't imagined. There was, Liz said, the stress and pressure of being in the limelight. Of being on display and looking—and being—optimistic and confident.

And Liz pointed out another disadvantage that became clear only toward the end of Alex's life, as recognition of Alex spread. "The lemonade stand," she said, "had become bigger than Alex." Toward the end, it got so that the stand defined who she was. People became attached to her because of the stand and what she had accomplished. People would ask to have their pictures taken with her, people she didn't even know. Alex was gracious, they said, and agreed whenever she could. But it was as if people were imposing their own image of who she was. I thought, but didn't say, that at least that image was well deserved. And that it was the sort of image that many other people—much older, perhaps—would have envied.

Did that image affect their own memories of Alex, I asked? When they looked back, did they see the figure that the public saw? Or did they see a young girl trying to live a normal life that was choreographed first around her cancer and then around the publicity that her lemonade stands brought?

On one hand, they said, all of her fundraising was somewhat misleading. Jay pointed out that 95 percent of Alex's time was spent being a normal kid. A normal kid, he was quick to clarify, with a very serious illness. "The stand itself was not a huge part of what she was."

But perhaps it was. At the end of our conversation Liz admitted that she did think often about Alex's last months. "A lot of who a person is comes out in the last days," she observed. "Her last months say a lot about who she was, the kind of person she was. She was incredibly strong, incredibly dedicated, incredibly caring." So while the lemonade stand was not really a large part of Alex's identity, as Jay pointed out, it was nevertheless an illustration, or evidence, of the sort of child she was, and the sort of adult she would have become.

Imposing Meaning and Purpose

Ladislaw came back to the clinic two weeks later. Earlier that day I had checked with Peter O'Dwyer, an oncologist who runs early-phase trials at Penn, and with Amy Kramer, his clinic manager. They thought that there were several protocols that Ladislaw might be eligible for. "Might," because eligibility often hinges on a patient's functional status and on how severely his or her activity is limited. Ladislaw would have been eligible for the trials that Peter and Amy had in mind if his functional status was good enough. I thought it was, but functional status can change rapidly, and he might be much worse by the time Amy and Peter saw him.

Also, we all knew that functional status is in the eye of the beholder. Thinking of Ladislaw racing his daughter down the hall in clinic two weeks ago, I thought that, so far at least, his illness had had only a minor impact on his activity. On the scale that they used, the Eastern Cooperative Oncology Group scoring system, I thought that Ladislaw had a score of 1 (out of 4), indicating that his cancer had limited his activity in minor ways. But Amy and Peter might find deficits and limitations that I hadn't, and might give him a score of 2. He would be eligible for most protocols with my score of 1, but their score of 2 or more would exclude him from many. So Amy and Peter weren't able to tell me that Ladislaw would definitely be eligible, only that there were several possibilities.

As I got off the phone with them, I decided that even though I couldn't offer a trial that Ladislaw would definitely be eligible for, I would tell him what I could. So after I ushered Ladislaw and Emma back to the exam room, I told them first about the uncertainty of eligibility determinations, and then about the trials that we thought he might be eligible for. Although I expected another ferocious attack from Emma, she was strangely subdued. I learned later that her sister, the nurse, had told Emma about patients whose cancer had miraculously gone into remission in Phase I trials. And that she had suggested that the possibility of benefit was much greater than what Ladislaw's oncologist, or I, had led them to believe.

And so, much more quickly than I had hoped, we agreed on a plan. Ladislaw would make an appointment to meet with Peter and Amy the following week to see what trials, if any, were available. They would tell Ladislaw and Emma about the trials in detail and Ladislaw could make an informed decision.

We moved on to talk about his pain and to argue, again, about whether a long acting pain medication was preferable. I finally prevailed, conditionally.

"OK, a test," he said. "We will make a test."

Knowing that it often took an hour or two for our pharmacy to dispense new medications, I wrote out a prescription for long-acting morphine and suggested that Emma might want to take it to the pharmacy while her father and I finished up. This maneuver, finally, gave me a chance to ask Ladislaw why he was so intent on enrolling in a Phase I trial. Although he didn't remark on it, I'm certain that Ladislaw appreciated that this opportunity was due entirely to our pharmacy's inefficiency, which I know he had derided in many previous visits to his oncologist.

Emma left and we both looked at the grey metal door for a moment, afraid it was going to open. It didn't, and so I asked Ladislaw again to help me understand why he wanted to enroll in a Phase I trial. I told him that I would help to arrange the visit no matter what he said. And he didn't really have to explain anything to me. But I was curious. I used that word intentionally because I thought—correctly, as it turned out—that curiosity was a motivation that Ladislaw would both understand and respect.

He became animated, then, in the way that I remembered him in our first meeting. But more assured, almost professorial. He wasn't going to offer me an explanation, I realized, he was going to give me a lecture. No longer doctor and patient, we were now student and professor.

"Do you know the term 'kludge'?"

I wasn't sure I had heard him correctly. His East European accent was thin, and barely detectable most of the time. But it could be disorienting when his language strayed into new territory.

A kludge? I didn't.

A kludge, he explained, was an engineering term that described a collection of parts that are thrown together to get a job done. ("Kludge" was Ladislaw's spelling, written out with typically impatient haste on the back of an envelope, but I've also seen "kluge.") A kludge is an effective but inelegant solution to a problem. So to carry packages on a bicycle, he said, you might tie a basket to the handlebars with wire. You would need to keep it off the front wheel with a block of wood, and you'd have to wrap the whole mess with duct tape. The result was functional, but that was all.

He emphasized this point, stabbing at my knee with a long, bony forefinger. It had no "merit." It was a contraption that was not as effective as it could be, and uglier than it needed to be. It would probably satisfy someone, but would make an engineer wince. That, he said, was a kludge. He sat back in his chair, like a professor who has made a particularly important point and was generously giving his students a chance to write it down.

"What my dear daughter doesn't understand, is that my regimen of medications, tests, procedures, and so on is nothing but a kludge."

He went on to say that the days he could see stretching out in front of him had no structure, no purpose. His treatment regimen was a collection of medications, tests, procedures, and routines that had been assembled over time to achieve a variety of aims. He had received radiation therapy to the metastases in his lung and lymph nodes, for instance, and several forms of systemic chemotherapy, as well as his pain medication. Together, this haphazard collection of treatments was the medical equivalent of a basket tied to a bicycle. As inelegant, I suppose, and about as unstable.

As a patient who wanted to live, he recognized the value of each part of his regimen. But as an engineer accustomed to elegant solutions, he detested the complexity that the regimen required. He wanted, instead, a simple plan, whose parts were as stripped down as possible. The minimum needed to accomplish a goal.

He had given this a great deal of thought, he said, and he decided there was no way that a simple medication regimen could possibly be effective. He recognized the need for each of the medications and chemotherapy that he was receiving. Getting rid of some of them would be like peeling the duct tape or the string off the handlebar basket—the result would be marginally simpler, but also less effective.

If he couldn't simplify his treatment regimen, Ladislaw had decided, he would rethink the purpose of whatever time he had left. And the cleanest, simplest way he could see to use the time he had left was to enroll in a research study.

If that sounds coldly intellectual, remember, as I had to force myself to, that simplicity was what drove Ladislaw throughout his life. For him, engineering was less a profession than a religion. So a goal that might appear to be purely utilitarian was in fact a perfect expression of who he was.

This explanation helped me, finally, to understand Ladislaw's casual dismissal of the probability that he would benefit from participating in a trial. That possibility of benefit, and the consequent complexity of its trade-off against side effects, would have been distasteful. Instead, it was the simple equation of a Phase I trial—participation in exchange for future knowledge—that appealed to him.

He wanted the rest of his life to be useful. Not only to be useful, but useful in the right way. This brought an added appeal to his plan, I think, because Ladislaw believed that he was a perfect research subject. He was "so-so smart," he said with a mix of humor and genuine modesty. He thought like a scientist. And he could tell the researchers how well a drug was working. So he wasn't just looking for a purpose—any purpose. He was looking for something much more elusive—a purpose that fit perfectly with his talents and abilities.

The psychiatrist and Holocaust survivor Victor Frankl would have understood this, I think. After he was transferred to Dachau from Auschwitz, he was asked to volunteer in another camp where typhus patients were being quarantined. None of his friends who were physicians volunteered, and most advised him not to go. But, he says, he felt that he had to. He knew he would die soon, he wrote, but at least there would be some sense in his death if he were to die, as a physician, taking care of others. "I thought that it would doubtless be more to the purpose to try and help my comrades as a doctor than to vegetate or finally lose my life as the unproductive laborer that I was then. For me this was simple mathematics, not sacrifice."

Ladislaw the engineer no doubt would have appreciated Frankl's allusion to "simple mathematics." It is a phrase that seems to describe perfectly Ladislaw's own decision. It was as if he had spun through a series of complex calculations that were opaque to the rest of us, including Emma, and determined that enrolling in a Phase I trial was the correct solution.

But Ladislaw's motivation was more nuanced, too. For instance, those calculations also seemed to me to have an aesthetic context. To Ladislaw any simple answer, like a crisp blueprint or an elegant equation, was admirable, even beautiful. And, conversely, there was something fundamentally distasteful and ugly about parts that were out of place, thrown together in a "kludge." So I think his choice to enroll in a Phase I trial was also guided by a sense of beauty and elegance.

Finally, I think that Ladislaw's motivation had moral roots as well. He seemed to believe—with a strength of feeling that could almost be called a religion—that there is a fundamental obligation to pursue the best possible use of things, and ourselves. One analogy he used in one of our conversations stuck with me. He became visibly disturbed as he talked about how one of his cancer treatments was akin to using a monkey wrench as a hammer to loosen a bolt. It wasn't just that this particular use—or misuse—of the tool was inefficient. More than that, it was somehow morally offensive, as if he saw such misuse as a visible symptom of a deeper character weakness.

So Ladislaw's choice to be "useful" was really, I think, no more "simple mathematics" than Frankl's was. Or if it was such a thing, then it also seems true that for Ladislaw "simple mathematics" is a thing of beauty, and that to follow its guidance is a moral obligation.

In a sense, they were both trying to wrest some sort of meaning, some purpose, from a death that was in most respects illogical and unfair. By participating in research, Ladislaw felt he had a chance to impose a purpose not just on his last months, but on the illness itself. It would be a rare bit of good fortune that his cancer—otherwise senseless and without logic—afflicted him, someone who was ideally suited to participate in a trial, and to learn something from it.

I don't mean that Ladislaw interpreted this turn of events in some teleological sense. He was not particularly spiritual, as far as I know, and I don't think he believed that his cancer came to him as part of some grand plan. But I do think that Ladislaw saw an opportunity to impose his own purpose. Just as he used his stint in the Army as a maintenance worker to redesign kitchen equipment, he would use this experience with cancer to learn, to teach, and to improve. This was the purpose that his cancer offered, a chance to impose structure on his last days, and a chance to make his death "count."

Ladislaw

As I expected, Ladislaw wasn't eligible for any Phase I trial. The combination of his increasing frailty and fatigue, as well as new problems, like mild kidney failure, made him ineligible for all of the protocols that were open. Ladislaw did find a trial in New York City for which he might be eligible. But the train trip proved to be more than he could manage.

That bounding restless energy that I first saw in our waiting room had disappeared, and even getting to the train station on the morning of his appointment was a challenge. He and Emma sat on one of the hard wooden benches in Philadelphia's 30th Street Station, waiting for Ladislaw to gather the energy to walk down the steps to the train. But as their train arrived and left, they sat there. It became clear that Ladislaw simply didn't have the strength to travel, let alone to convince the doctors in New York that he would be the ideal research subject that he had imagined he could be.

I didn't see Ladislaw again after that failed trip to New York. I was in touch with Emma for a time—weekly, for a while—until Ladislaw enrolled in a hospice program several weeks later. He died, I heard, in the hospice's inpatient unit about six months after I met him.

I was disappointed to hear that he was never able to enroll in a trial, of course, because I knew how much it meant to him. Mostly, though, I was relieved that he wouldn't have to face the hassles and indignities of participating in a trial. And I was relieved, too, because I simply didn't see that participating in a Phase I trial was the natural, perfect choice that Ladislaw seemed to think it was. Not all such studies are valuable, for instance, and many of them never produce data that can be translated into improved treatment. Indeed, I often wonder how much of the effort—of investigators and research subjects—ends up in a wastebasket. And the results of many trials simply offer more evidence, as if any were needed, that cancer is a particularly virulent enemy and that there are no silver bullets. And so I was skeptical that a Phase I trial truly offered the chance to be useful that Ladislaw said he wanted.

Oddly, Ladislaw didn't seem to recognize the possibility that his participation in a trial might not offer the benefits to others that he had hoped. That blind spot was, and is, surprising to me, given the intensity with which he scrutinized the idea of participating. He seemed to have examined these trials closely and carefully, just as he might have searched for flaws in, say, a bridge or a building's foundation. And there were many aspects of them that Ladislaw did appreciate, such as the lack of potential benefit, for instance, and the possibility of side effects. Yet this was one that he missed. Perfectly willing to assume that there was no chance that he himself would benefit, Ladislaw seemed oddly unable to recognize that a trial he participated in might be unsuccessful and that no one else would benefit, either.

I'm still not sure why Ladislaw's gimlet-eyed scrutiny—otherwise quite thorough—missed this flaw. Perhaps he took the view that it was his intention that "counted," and that his time would be well spent if his intent, at least, was to be useful. For someone else, this might have been a plausible interpretation. But Ladislaw was nothing if not a hardheaded utilitarian, and I suspect he would pay only scant attention to intentions. So perhaps he was motivated by faith in the scientific method, faith that even if a trial did not identify an effective drug, this failure would, somehow, contribute to medical science.

Whatever the reason, for Ladislaw enrolling in a trial was a way of guaranteeing that his last months would make a contribution. Enrolling in a Phase I trial was, perhaps, a "safe" choice. "Safe" in the sense that, at least as Ladislaw saw it, his time would be well utilized. He would be "useful."

NINE

Jose

Hopelessness and Fear

Although a few of the stories in this book are inspirational accounts of what people have done with the time they had left, almost all offer excruciating reminders that they could have done more. These stories are questions, in a sense. What might these people have done if only they'd been given more time—more time to decide what was important, more time to choose, and more time to act? But for a few people, like Jose, even the time they have is too much.

Jose

Jose wasn't Hispanic, despite the way his name was written. Short for Joseph, he pronounced it with one syllable, as in "rose." Jose was African-American, in his forties, and had hepatitis C and hepatocellular (liver) cancer. His cancer was quite advanced and had been causing severe pain for more than a month before I met him. But Jose also had a long history of abusing drugs, including heroin and prescription medications, and that made his physicians uneasy about prescribing opioids. His doctor wouldn't give Jose morphine unless he agreed to live in a nursing home where, she thought, the potential for drug abuse could be minimized. So Jose came to our palliative-care clinic at the Philadelphia VA hospital with severe pain that confined him to a wheelchair, cradling a jam jar half-full of acetaminophen.

When I first saw him in the corner of our waiting room, he was sitting in his wheelchair, with one heel and the other toe resting on the tile floor, as if in spring-loaded readiness for a pirouette. His face was drawn and jaundiced, and his skin was so light that he seemed depleted and insubstantial. Jose rested there with the distant, unfocused gaze of a subway rider wearing headphones, sunk in music that no one else can hear. He reclined in the wheelchair almost theatrically, leaning back with long sinewy arms draped over the armrests and delicate fingers like spider legs flicking an inaudible rhythm on the spokes of the wheels.

It's virtually impossible to look like anything other than an invalid while sitting alone in a wheelchair that has been shunted to the far corner of a crowded waiting room. But Jose seemed very much alive. More than that, he had style, a commodity that was in short supply in that particular waiting room. Jose even managed to wear his black Adidas track suit, which would have looked like a temporary costume on anyone else, with an almost formal elegance. I paused for a moment in the doorway before introducing myself, struck again by the grace and style that a few of my patients can summon when struggling with a degree of pain that would reduce most of us to the meanest level of existence.

I had no idea, as I watched Jose across the waiting room, that this would be virtually the only calm, peaceful moment that we would share. Developing a relationship proved to be frustratingly difficult, because the sense of style that I saw that day was joined to, and perhaps motivated by, a deep vein of self-contained independence. Jose had become resigned to expect very little, yet he was also convinced that what little he had could be taken from him all too easily. So Jose faced the world, the health care system, and me, with a sort of hopeless suspicion.

Developing a relationship was particularly difficult for me, the only physician in our palliative-care clinic. Jose's experiences with physicians up until that point had been disappointing, and his expectations of me were correspondingly low. And I'm afraid I did nothing to raise those expectations the day I met him.

He was worried that I might tell him to reduce his acetaminophen dose because it was damaging his liver. I did, because it was. And Jose, predictably, became angry and threatened to leave, which was a pattern that would be repeated numerous times in future visits. That exchange was not particularly productive.

More productive, though, was a longer discussion we had that first day about how we could manage Jose's pain without sending him to a nursing home. This, it turned out, was his primary concern. Although he had had long-term relationships with both men and women, he was currently single and lived alone in an apartment in West Philadelphia. Until his pain had confined him to his apartment, he had enjoyed an active social life, centered mostly on bars, clubs, and block parties in the neighborhood. And he had absolutely no intention of giving this social life up permanently to go live in a nursing home room next to, as he put it, "some old brain-dead piece of meat rotting on a piss-soaked mattress." He wrinkled his nose as he said this, as if he could smell that mattress. When I thought about it for a moment, I realized that I could, too.

Although there are many nursing homes that are quite good, Jose succeeded in fixing that image so clearly in my own mind that I promised him that we would do whatever we could to help him stay at home. So over the next month or two, we saw him every week in clinic. And with the help of Nancy Wiedemer, a nurse practitioner who is very skilled at managing pain in patients with a history of drug use, we got him on a regimen of methadone for his pain. (Methadone is actually a very effective opioid or "narcotic" analgesic, but it doesn't produce the euphoria of other opioids and therefore it has no abuse potential itself.) Within a few days, the methadone had controlled Jose's pain well enough that he could get around as much as he needed to, so he could sleep at night, and so he could begin to reconstruct a social life.

But our clinic team—Jack Coffey, Lucy Pierre, Priscilla Kissick—and I began to realize that we had traded one problem for another. That we had controlled his pain without having to place him in a nursing home was a substantial victory, and gained us Jose's trust. However, Jose was still in his home alone, with a prognosis of probably not more than three or four months.

This was a problem because we all saw quite clearly that even though his pain was well controlled, other problems—fatigue, shortness of breath, fluid retention—would soon appear. Jose would grow weaker, making it increasingly difficult for him to come to clinic, to go shopping, to see his friends, and to care for himself at home. Eventually, the cancer that was spreading throughout his liver might also cause confusion and delirium—common effects of poor liver function—that would make it impossible for him to stay at home safely. When that happened, there were no family members who could care for him at home, and we would be forced to place him in a nursing home.

As we expected, after two good months during which Jose seemed to get much of his energy back, his condition began to deteriorate. He began to miss his clinic appointments, and when he did come in, he seemed increasingly fragile and exhausted. He was always in good spirits and never admitted to feeling sad or depressed. But the style and grace that were so obvious on his first visit were gone, replaced by a kind of gentle endurance.

In retrospect, I think that Jose's fatigue was due only partly to his advancing cancer. In addition, I suspect that he had also begun to see the trajectory of his illness just as clearly as we had when we first met him. And I imagine that this knowledge was at least as mentally debilitating as his cancer was physically draining.

Eventually, when Jose had missed several appointments in a row, we calculated that he had almost run out of methadone and that he would need a refill to avoid withdrawal. Our pharmacy and the postal service, we knew, would never get a delivery to him in time. So that afternoon in the clinic conference room, Jack and Lucy looked at me expectantly.

They knew that I had made home visits in the past, sometimes sneaking out of clinic when things were slow. What they didn't know was that I made those visits as much for my own mental health as for our patients' benefit. Those were difficult times for me, in many ways. I was still early in a research career at a competitive Ivy League medical school, where expectations for "productivity" (papers, presentations, and large research grants) were ambitious. Those of us who joined the faculty knew that we had only a few short years either to produce or leave. I hoped to be in the former category but suspected that I was destined for the latter. It was a relief to be able to forget about the pile of rejection letters for papers and research grants on my desk, at least for a while. So I would make home visits whenever I could, escaping the hospital and academic world for an hour at a time to concentrate on one patient's problems. The first and last visit I made to Jose's apartment was one of these.

Early that afternoon I set off on foot into West Philadelphia, which was at the time one of the worst neighborhoods in the city. Mercifully, Jose lived close to the hospital, just a few blocks beyond the outer ring of the most adventurous Penn faculty homes. As I walked up the front path to the large brick Victorian where Jose had a third-floor apartment, I saw a heavyset woman who must have been his landlady, sitting on a rickety porch swing that swayed precariously under her considerable weight. We knew each other, in a way. Jose's phone had been cut off a few months earlier, so we'd been calling his landlady with messages and to schedule his appointments.

No, she hadn't seen him that day, which wasn't unusual. He often stayed up late, listening to old gospel records whose sounds would drift down softly and through her open windows. The Blue Ridge Quartet, I imagined, and Jack Holcomb, and the White Sisters. I knew these names from our conversations in clinic. As I was filling out his new prescriptions, Jose would describe yet another group, and would tell me what made them unique and how each had contributed to all of the music that had come since.

Jose's landlady said she'd walk up with me ("to check on my boy," her only tenant) but then, perhaps thinking of the two long flights of stairs, she simply pointed the way and settled back on the long-suffering porch swing. The house was dark and dense, cooler than the humid August air on the porch, but dirtier too, with a heavy smell of onions and wax and mothballs. I felt like an intruder as I climbed the long straight set of stairs that led up from the front hallway, not sure whether to trust the creaking stairs beneath me or the banister that gave a little under my right hand like a loose tooth. Actually, I had little confidence in either once I'd seen the landlady's massive daybed in the front room. If she slept on the first floor, I realized, it was entirely possible that Jose (about 120 pounds) and I (not much more) were the only ones who had used this staircase in a very long time.

The gloom became almost complete when I reached the second-floor landing. I swept my hand along the wall hoping for a light switch but succeeded only in dislodging a picture. Ignoring the grit on the floor that was probably the remnants of the picture's glass, I rehung it by feel and moved on blindly. Turning the corner for the last flight of stairs, I was met by a peel of light from beneath the door at the top of the stairs that was blinding at first but which offered just enough light to guide me up the stairs.

The artificial midnight in the stairwell made me forget for a moment that it was a sunny summer afternoon. I knocked softly at first, as a late-night visitor might. There was no answer and I knocked harder, calling Jose's name and my own.

Like some Raymond Chandler denouement, the partly sprung latch gave way and the thick wooden door swung open several inches, blinding me completely, again. As I called out Jose's name three or four times, my eyes adjusted and I could make out Jose's feet, crossed in bedroom slippers, framed by the underside of the table at which he was sitting.

But long past the point that Philip Marlowe would have noticed that Jose's feet hadn't responded to my crescendo of calls, I hovered at the door and leaned in over the threshold as if, somehow, that would help me to get Jose's attention. Eventually, though, I pushed through the door and into the room to find Jose sitting in an armchair pulled up to an old white kitchen table with chipped enamel that could have served as a desk and dining table, head resting on crossed arms. He might have been taking a nap. But he wasn't.

He was wearing a cheap pair of headphones that had slipped partway off his ears. They were connected to a portable CD player on the table in front of him, and the escaping sounds of music sounded harsh, gritty, what I recognized only much later as the hymn "The Old Rugged Cross." I stood there for a few moments, and as the song ended and another begun, I realized then that Jose had set the CD player to repeat the same song over and over. And then I realized that he was dead.

Feeling a bit like a medical student again—it's remarkable how thin that veneer of training really is when we're caught by surprise—I tried to shake Jose awake. I summarily concluded he was dead, forgetting the usual maneuvers that we use to pronounce death such as checking for breathing or a pulse. I turned to move toward the door, but paused. It felt wrong—disrespectful, somehow—to leave a dead body unattended. Caught by this feeling at the top of the stairs, I hesitated. Then, as a compromise, I opened the door wide, as if doing so would somehow fulfill my obligation, and made my way carefully back down the stairs.

Jose's landlady didn't seem particularly surprised when I told her what I'd found. From the messages that she relayed, she'd probably assembled a reasonably accurate picture of Jose's health. And so she reached behind her swing for the phone and called the police. With surprisingly little preamble (had she done this before?) she was explaining the situation. After the initial introductions, we passed the phone back and forth like a comfortably married couple sharing news with grandchildren. No, she had heard no sign of a disturbance. Yes, I could affirm that he was terminally ill. No, he had no close friends. In the end, I suspect that it was my information that Jose had advanced cancer that offered the final necessary reassurance that this was a natural death, and which avoided paramedics, police, and neighbors.

But I wasn't entirely comfortable with that explanation as I threaded my way back to Penn's campus over sidewalks cracked and heaved with neglect. What could have caused a sudden death? Sudden, that is, without symptoms that would have led Jose to seek attention? Increased pain, or bleeding, or fever signaling an infection would have prompted Jose to call us, I was sure.

Although I was puzzled, I didn't begin to suspect that Jose might have taken his own life until his landlady called me about a week later. She and her daughter had been cleaning out Jose's apartment and they'd found a small amount of leftover methadone from the VA. She was wondering what she should do with it. In the course of that conversation, she also mentioned that she found several other pill bottles that were empty.

As far as I knew, Jose was getting all of his medications from us, so I was skeptical at first. But his landlady was adamant. Lined up neatly next to Jose's bathroom sink were five non-VA medication bottles, and she read the labels haltingly, word by word. Four were for opioids like morphine and oxycodone, and one was for lorazepam, a sedative. They were from four different physicians, none of whom I knew. All of the prescriptions had been filled within the last two months, but the patient names on the bottles were different. So Jose had either used an alias to get prescriptions from other physicians (unlikely) or he had bought the pills on the street. And he had done so, and used them all, in a short period of time.

Recognizing Suicide Near the End of Life

Did Jose take his own life? Lucy, Jack, Priscilla, Nancy, and I couldn't agree. The suddenness of his death, the way the CD player was left on, and the medications all suggested to me that he might have. But the others weren't sure. Jose had no signs of depression, they said, and was still able to live at home, independently, so why would he take his life now?

I wasn't convinced by their version, but neither was I particularly convincing in presenting my own. Perhaps I didn't really want to be arguing the side that I found myself on. I didn't want to believe that Jose had committed suicide any more than my colleagues did.

Our reluctance was not really surprising. Those of us who take care of people near the end of life are loath to recognize suicide among our patients because suicide is often a signal that we've failed. Most of us assume, at some level, that suffering is an underlying motivation for suicide. And since our primary task, and often our only task, is to relieve suffering, we're particularly likely to interpret a patient's suicide as our failure. So suicide is something we cannot afford to let ourselves notice too often.

In addition, though, this reluctance to recognize suicide is also the result of a scarcity of information. For instance, the facts that we hear about the end of a patient's life are often incomplete or ambiguous or both. A hospice nurse might visit the home of a patient who has just died and find that all of the patient's morphine—what should have been several weeks' worth—is missing. Perhaps that patient took an overdose, but perhaps a family member used it. Or, most likely, the patient simply had increased pain and used up the morphine more rapidly than the nurse expected. In cases like these, we simply don't know whether a patient took his own life. In fact, there are very few instances in which I'm sure that a patient I cared for committed suicide. One or two, perhaps, over the past ten years.

Finally, I think that those of us who work exclusively with the dying fail to recognize suicides because it's often hard for us to appreciate the motivations of people who choose to end their lives. Our work demands that we try to imagine the potential that each day holds, and that process of imagination lets us create "good days" for people who are a week away from death. We even say that a patient had a "good death," a term that many find odd and slightly ghoulish. Within this frame of reference, in which even the last hours of a patient's life can offer rewards of meaning, satisfaction, and growth, it's difficult for us to appreciate what might lead a patient to commit suicide.

This combination of uncertainty and an almost willful blindness toward suicide made it difficult for all of us to consider Jose's possible motivations honestly. We had treated his pain and he had a few months ahead. So why might he have wanted to take his own life?

Assisted Suicide

In order to understand why someone like Jose might take his own life, it's helpful, at least as a starting point, to find a set of circumstances in which suicide has been defined and painstakingly described. The best example, by a wide margin, is the practice known as physician-assisted suicide (PAS). The term PAS is used to refer to those instances in which a health care provider—usually a physician—provides a patient with the means to commit suicide. As I write this in 2009, PAS is permitted in The Netherlands, Belgium, Switzerland, and in the United States in Oregon and Washington.

How common is PAS? The uncomfortable truth is that no one really knows. Of course, we do know how often patients use PAS through legal mechanisms. In Oregon, for instance, only about thirty or so patients are reported to use PAS each year. The real question, though, is how common PAS is overall, if you count all those situations in which physicians provide some degree of assistance. One national survey found that about 3 percent of physicians had done this at least once. And this figure may be even higher—

about 11 percent in one study—among oncologists. These numbers are small, but they're not insignificant.

Furthermore, these numbers may actually underestimate the true incidence of PAS. Anthony Back, an oncologist, found that physicians may aid patients in committing suicide in small, hidden ways, by providing an extra prescription or a hint that a particular drug could be fatal if taken in an overdose. What is particularly interesting about Back's study is that although sometimes physicians know that they are giving these hints, often, it seems, they do not. So PAS may be more common than even physicians realize and more frequent, therefore, than they report.

We also know that many patients with serious illnesses think about ending their lives. In a survey, Zeke and Linda Emanuel found that about 10 percent of terminally ill patients said they were considering the possibility of suicide. When the Emanuels went back to those patients several months later, they found that many who had considered suicide no longer did, while others who had not previously considered suicide had begun to. So the number of people who think about committing suicide during the course of a terminal illness is likely to be much larger than a single survey would suggest.

Together, these results suggest that some patients with serious illnesses will consider suicide. If a typical oncologist, for instance, sees ten patients in a day, it's likely that at least one of them is thinking about suicide. Moreover, because people's feelings about suicide seem to change over time, a much larger number, maybe as many as three or four out of ten, have thought about suicide in the past, or will in the future.

In part because of these statistics, very few bioethics debates in recent history have raised as much energy and anger as the discussion about PAS has. In fact, disagreements about PAS have polarized many groups in law and ethics, and particularly those, like me, who care for patients near the end of life. I have many friends and colleagues in the field who have become distant, even cold, with one another because of this debate. PAS is one of those moral-ethical issues, like abortion, that is cruelly divisive.

Clarifying the ethics of PAS is not our task here. Nevertheless, the debate that has swirled around PAS has led to a great deal of discussion, reflection, and empirical research. So we know quite a bit about suicide in the setting of terminal illness. Therefore, PAS offers a unique opportunity to understand the motivations of people with serious illnesses who choose to end their own lives.

Suffering

There is a common belief that patients who are terminally ill take their own lives in order to relieve intractable suffering. It's a reasonable belief, or at least an understandable one. We are, most of us, all too aware of the sources of suffering—pain, shortness of breath, nausea—that come with advanced illness. And most of us have had experience with at least some of these symptoms. They're what we know and, therefore, they're what we know to be afraid of.

But is suffering really a common motivation for suicide among patients with terminal illness? There is some evidence to suggest that it is. Diane Meier, a palliative-care physician and geriatrician, conducted a survey of physicians in the United States and found that the most common motivation for suicide their patients reported was suffering associated with physical discomfort. Although Diane's is an important study, we need to remember that these motivations reflect physician's recollections. That is, they were not patients' reports of their motivations, but rather the motivations that physicians perceived. This distinction is important because physicians are arguably better able to detect physical symptoms than they are to recognize, say, undefined fear of the future or unfocused anxiety. So it is possible that the physicians in that study simply reported the motivations that they were able to recognize.

It's also important to keep in mind that actual suffering may be accompanied by, and overshadowed by, a fear of suffering in the future. Bob Pearlman, a geriatrician at the University of Washington, found that approximately two-thirds of requests for assistance in dying were motivated by a fear of suffering. Indeed, other very carefully designed studies of PAS requests in Oregon have found that requests are less likely to be motivated by actual suffering than by a fear of suffering in the future.

Although a fear of suffering is prominent in requests for PAS, I came to recognize it much later than I should have, when I was a palliative-care fellow at the University of Pennsylvania. That fellowship was, in many ways, a daunting learning experience. Although I was a board-certified internist and had taught residents and medical students, that fellowship threw me back on the steep end of the learning curve. And so for the first months in particular, I was Janet Abrahm's near-constant shadow, following her lead and watching patient consultations and family meetings unfold with a sense of wonder and disorientation that I hadn't felt since medical school.

It was one of the first consultations of my fellowship, when I was most unsteady, that Janet and I went together to see a woman in her early fifties who had ovarian cancer. We, or rather Janet, led the conversation. She assessed the woman's symptoms, talked with her about her goals for care, and arranged for a hospice visit. As we were standing to leave, though, the woman caught hold of the sleeve of my lab coat, holding me in place as Janet glided out the door.

"What is it going to be like?" she asked.

Janet had led the entire discussion to that point and was obviously in charge. Yet it seemed like this question was directed at me. And I had no idea what she meant.

But she obviously wanted an answer. More than that, she needed an answer. And she had to have one before she would let us—me—leave. Her grip had shifted from my sleeve to my forearm and showed no sign of loosening.

But what did she mean? And what was 'it'?

I looked to Janet in what had become, between us, an all-too-familiar call for a lifeline. And so Janet sat back down on the edge of the bed, I perched again on my chair, and Janet's face took on that beatific expression that she got sometimes in intense conversations with patients. Peaceful and comforting, it was the sort of expression that inspired patients to say whatever was on their minds, often surprising us and, occasionally, themselves.

What our patient wanted to know, Janet realized, was what dying would be like. Before answering, though, Janet found out what the woman was afraid of, and what her preconceptions were, and then offered reassurance that was tailored to those fears. And in a conversation that has played out dozens of times for me since then, our patient told Janet what she was afraid dying might be like. That it would be uncomfortable, with pain and nausea. And that it would be frightening, like a nightmare. Janet was able to reassure her not by categorical statements, but by describing the sorts of things that might happen, and what we would do to alleviate any suffering that might occur. In the years since that conversation, Janet's careful balance between asking questions and offering reassurance has been a sort of template, or guide, that I've tried to follow with my own patients.

Somewhere in that conversation the woman's grip on my arm relaxed, and her hand came to rest gently on my arm. Her expression changed, too, as if Janet had released a spring that had kept her wound up throughout our previous conversation. It was the first time in the hour or so that we had been in the room that she looked truly comfortable.

Up until that question, and Janet's gentle response, I had never given a moment's thought to the fears that we have about dying. A fear *of* dying, of course. And a corresponding desire to live. But not fears about what the process of dying would be like.

Once I started paying attention, though, I started seeing these fears in many of the patients I cared for. I met a man with lung cancer, for instance, who was afraid that the experience of dying would recapitulate the terrifying sensation he once had of waking up at the end of a surgical procedure, fully awake and able to feel but unable to move. And I met an older woman with advanced heart failure and near-constant shortness of breath who dreaded the sensation of suffocation that she believed would press down on her during her final hours. And I've met many patients—far too many—who were so afraid of dying in pain that they hoarded their pain medications to make sure that they would have enough when they needed them most.

When I teach medical students and nursing students, I try to portray these fears as symptoms, like pain or nausea, that they have an obligation to identify and treat. I don't mean to simplify or medicalize what are, really, complex sources of suffering. Instead, my point is that just as doctors and nurses have an obligation to recognize and treat suffering, they have an obligation to address fears of suffering.

My students often remain unconvinced. Fears of death are entirely rational, they say. Of course death is terrifying. Who wouldn't be afraid?

In these conversations, though, I've noticed that they tend to project their own fears onto others. They themselves are afraid of dying, and therefore fear must be normal, and perhaps even universal. And so in an effort to try to help them to look at those fears in a more objective way, without filtering them through their own conceptions of what dying will be like, I tell them about a story of suicide in circumstances that none of them is likely to experience.

There is a startling exhibit in London's Imperial War Museum that is as remarkable a story of survival as it is of suicide. Prominently displayed in the museum is a photograph of two men, emaciated to the point of death, one of whom is in a wheelchair on what appears to be a wide veranda. At least one of the men seems to be speaking, and they are attended by a well-dressed man and woman who appear to be listening carefully, almost worshipfully. The caption identifies the standing couple as the Duke and Duchess of Windsor and the seated men only as Roy Widdicombe and Robert

Tapscott, "after their ordeal." That description, I was to learn, is a perfect example of quintessentially British understatement.

On the night of August 20, 1940, in the South Atlantic, the British merchant ship *Anglo-Saxon* was sunk by the German ship *Widder*. Only one lifeboat was spared, which carried the seven survivors (out of a crew of forty-one): Francis Penny, a gunner; Roy Pilcher, a radio operator; Leslie Morgan, the assistant cook; Roy Widdicombe and Bob Tapscott, both able seamen; Lionel Hawks, the third engineer; and Barry Denny, the first mate. The following morning, the lifeboat was alone on a calm sea, with no other ship in sight, little food, and almost no water. Roy Pilcher died a few days later, of gangrene from a foot wound he had suffered during the attack, setting the stage for what could have been a classic drama of resistance and survival.

But it was Francis Penny, on the fourteenth day, who altered the plot of the story that would unfold. Although Penny, too, had a leg wound, it did not seem to be life-threatening. Yet on the fourteenth day, he simply stepped off the stern of the lifeboat and allowed himself to float away.

The remaining men were profoundly affected by what they felt sure was his suicide. In an instant, he had demonstrated how easily, and quickly, their suffering could be ended. And that afternoon, the desultory talk among the men turned to the example that Penny's death had given them, and what a death by drowning would be like, and whether it would be better or worse than a slow death due to thirst.

The next morning, their meager supply of water gone, Barry Denny broke the silence and announced he was going to follow Penny over the side. Lionel Hawks said he would join him, but only if Denny would help him. And so Hawks had a "last meal" of ship's biscuit and saltwater, Denny gave his signet ring to Widdicombe to give to Denny's mother, the men shook hands all around, and Denny and Hawks stepped off the stern of the lifeboat holding tightly to each other. The note in the boat's log that day is terse: "Chief mate and 3rd Engineer go over the side no water."

Leslie Morgan died four days later, leaving only Widdicombe and Tapscott, alone after almost three weeks in an open boat and almost a week without water. What followed was a strange ballet as Widdicombe and Tapscott alternately considered and rejected the option of suicide. They left a note and slipped over the side, but Widdicombe scrambled back over the gunwale, and after a moment's hesitation Tapscott followed. Widdicombe was not yet ready to die, and Tapscott was not ready to die alone. Several hours later this scene was repeated, leaving them clinging to the boat. They decided, finally, that they could not bring themselves to die yet. Both were eventually rescued weeks later. (Roy Widdicombe died a short time later in another ship sunk by a German U-boat. Bob Tapscott survived the war but led a solitary life with chronic depression. When he died suddenly in 1963, his death was ruled a suicide.) And so of the seven men who survived the *Anglo-Saxon*'s sinking, three chose death rather than further suffering and two came very close.

Whenever I tell students this story, there's something about it that seems to capture not just their attention, but also their imagination. Perhaps it's simply the drama of uncertainty that the narrative creates. Who will live and who won't? It is, after all, an adventure story, which is a genre whose rarity in our medical school curriculum gives it a certain appeal.

But the meaning that this story has for me—and the lesson I try to share with my students—is that the lifeboat's atmosphere of unrestrained fear and uncertainty is not unlike what many of our patients experience. It's more extreme, of course. But that's what gives this story its weight and impact, transforming it into an allegory. I warn my students that the fear that ran rampant in that small lifeboat, taking the lives of people who might otherwise have survived, serves as a vivid illustration of the fear that can overwhelm our patients when we fail to provide enough guidance and support.

This was a fear that Jose may have shared. He had lived through several months of debilitating pain before he came to our clinic, negotiating and pleading unsuccessfully for pain medications. Jose was more acutely aware than most patients are that only a physician's signature on a prescription pad preserved the fragile balance of comfort that he had achieved.

Of course, I hope that he trusted us to provide him with the pain medications that he needed. And that he knew that we would do our best to ensure his comfort. Still, he had been disappointed by health care providers in the past, and there is really no reason to believe that Jose would have placed his complete trust in us.

Control and Dignity

Perhaps I could have done a better job of reassuring Jose that we would do our best to control his pain. Indeed, in most cases, I feel that I *can* reassure my patients who are afraid of suffering. I can't promise that they won't feel any discomfort at all, but I can promise that the discomfort they feel won't be more than they can manage. More important, I can promise to stay with them and to work through symptoms they have and new problems that arise. In my experience, that last point is sometimes the only reassurance that they need.

What I can't guarantee is that my patients will be able to live independently and autonomously. Or that they will retain control over their thinking and actions. Or that they will continue to be the people that they have always been.

It often seems to me that this is what many of my patients want more than anything else. In fact, in several studies of PAS, a loss of independence and dignity are among the most prominent motivations for requests for assistance in dying. For instance, Linda Ganzini found that three of the most common reasons for PAS requests were a loss of independence, a fear of losing independence, and a need for control.

To fully appreciate the significance of this result, it helps to understand how most chronic illnesses progress. Think of the most common causes of death in industrialized countries—heart disease, lung disease, cancer, and dementia. For all of these, advancing illness will limit our ability to perform the "activities of daily living" that we take for granted, like washing, eating, and using the toilet. The result, for many of us, will be a series of losses that will progressively constrict our ability to live independently.

In a wonderfully elegant study, June Lunney, a nurse researcher, looked carefully at the level of function of about 4,000 patients in their last year of life. She found that some patients with chronic progressive illnesses like dementia were dependent in virtually all activities of daily living in their last months. Others, like those with heart failure or lung disease, were dependent only in some. But one of the most interesting findings was that even those patients who died suddenly (e.g., of a massive heart attack or stroke) had difficulty with at least one activity of daily living before they died. So almost all of us, no matter how we die, can expect some decline in our ability to function independently. We will need to rely on others—friends, family members, or professional caregivers—to help us in and out of bed, to bathe us, and to feed us.

That is a natural and expected part of dying, yet it's something that many people find frightening. I made a home visit once to an elderly woman with severe heart failure because our hospice team was concerned that she wasn't able to live independently anymore. But Myrna was furiously resistant to all of our suggestions that she move to her son's home in the suburbs. "I'd rather die," she told us with a ferocious intensity. "If you send me there, I'll wait till no one's looking and I'll walk outside"—this was in January—"and I'll freeze myself to death before anyone notices I'm gone."

She was fiercely independent. She had been a successful businesswoman for most of her life and was unaccustomed to relying on others—even her children—for anything. She was "making do," Myrna told the hospice nurse. Moreover, she already had everything that she needed, and she had more help in her apartment than she could possibly get at her son's house.

We were skeptical. We knew that her heart failure had severely curtailed her ability to walk, and we couldn't understand how an elderly woman who became short of breath moving from her bed to a chair could possibly live independently. We thought it was obvious that her situation would be improved if she were to live with her son and daughter-in-law.

So I went to visit Myrna in her apartment one afternoon and spent a futile hour trying to convince her that a move would give her additional assistance. She would be able to do more, I told her, and she would enjoy a better quality of life. The choice seemed logical to me, but Myrna rejected all my arguments.

I had all but given up when she excused herself for a moment and rose unsteadily from her recliner, waving away my offers of help. She began to make her way, painfully slowly, toward the bathroom about 20 feet away. Within a few steps she became visibly short of breath. Fending off my renewed offers of support, she pivoted with a heavy grace and sank onto a rather uncomfortable-appearing wooden armchair with the Penn logo that, fortunately, had been next to her just when it seemed she couldn't take another step.

I hovered next to her with a sort of embarrassed superiority, smug but also sad that I had been proven right. I noticed, though, that she seemed undaunted. She rested for a moment and then rose, making her teetering way back through the apartment. Again, though, just as it seemed that she would collapse into the thick carpet at her feet, Myrna turned and lowered herself into another chair that seemed to be in just the right place.

I realized, then, that the appearance of these chairs was not the lucky accident that it had seemed, but rather the result of careful planning. These chairs were her way stations, their precise positions calibrated to within a foot or so. And they'd probably inched closer together, week by week, as her illness progressed.

A few moments later, as Myrna disappeared and the bathroom

door clicked shut, I decided that she really was "making do." She had assembled a series of props and supports that allowed her to be independent, albeit within tight constraints. She could get around her own apartment and, we later learned, she had carefully choreographed the roles of several neighbors who helped with shopping. In fact, she had even arranged for her longtime hairdresser to make home visits. She'd done all of this to preserve her independence as long as possible.

In the end, Myrna's family was able to ensure that she could continue to live in her apartment until she died. It's true that she became increasingly weak and came to require someone—her son, her daughter-in-law, or a hired nurse—in the apartment with her virtually around the clock. Indeed, soon she had all the help that she would have received at her son's home. But she was in her home, and could arrange her life along the lines to which she had become accustomed. She died about a month after I met her, at home, in her sleep.

Although Myrna didn't commit suicide in order to maintain control over her life, there are many others who have. And these examples are not limited to people with chronic illnesses. For instance, embedded throughout the persecutions that swept thought Europe from the 1940s through the 1960s are countless stories of those who took their own lives. These stories emerged from the Holocaust first, but later from the labor camps of Eastern Europe and from the Soviet gulag. Although the circumstances of each death were different, fear, uncertainty, and a progressive erosion of control and dignity led many people to take their own lives.

In one account, Alexander Donat, a Holocaust survivor, writes angrily of the suicides that he witnessed during the September 1942 campaign that engulfed the Warsaw Ghetto, where he was living with his wife, Lena, and son, Wlodek. For Donat, the possibility of suicide offered insurance, of a sort—insurance that they could take control over whatever time they had left. He describes, for instance, the cyanide pills they carried as their "most precious treasure," and as their "final bulwark of hope."

And sometimes motivations of dignity and control are mixed with defiance. When Polina Melnikova hung herself in the Siberian Kolyma work camp, her friend Evgenia Ginzburg reported, as a sort of epitaph, that Melnikova "had asserted her rights to be a person by acting as she had, and she had made an efficient job of it." The historian and literary theorist Tzvetan Todorov, too, suggests that a desire for suicide in those camps was often a defiant attempt to control one's life. "By committing suicide," he wrote, "one alters the course of events—if only of the last time in one's life—instead of simply reacting to them. Suicides of this kind are acts of defiance, not desperation."

Although these sentiments were expressed under very different circumstances than those that Jose faced, I think that they could apply equally well. For instance, Jose's fears of being sent to a nursing home were never far below the surface of our conversations. He must have thought about suicide as a way—perhaps the only way that he could see—of avoiding the indignity of living and dying in a nursing home. And Jose's attitude throughout the time that I knew him was nothing if not defiant. He had been told repeatedly over the past few months what he could and couldn't do, so his death was, perhaps, his last opportunity to arrange his life as he wanted it to be.

Fear of Becoming a Burden

For many of my patients, what appears to be a desire for control is, at least in part, motivated by a fear of becoming a burden to others. Sometimes that fear has sufficient potency to motivate thoughts of suicide. Not long ago, I was visiting a hospice to check on the progress of a research project. I'd taken a taxi from my hotel early in the morning and found the offices quiet and subdued. There were hushed, almost furtive conversations among two or three people in corners, but the frenetic energy that typically overtakes a busy hospice on a Monday morning was missing.

It turned out that one of their patients had committed suicide the night before outside a nearby emergency room. It wasn't only Michael's suicide, though, that disturbed the hospice staff, but the manner in which he carried it out. Apparently, he had left his house in the middle of the night while his wife was still asleep, taking only his wallet and a loaded shotgun. He had driven past the emergency room at the small community hospital in which he was known as a patient, and stopped instead at a larger hospital to which he had never been.

According to the police reconstruction of what transpired that night, Michael parked his car, got out, locked the doors, and walked to the hospital entrance, where he found an unattended wheelchair. He then walked to the concrete apron just beyond the light from the emergency room doors and sat in the wheelchair, placing his wallet and car keys on the concrete in front of him. He locked the chair's wheels against the shotgun's recoil, and shot himself.

Michael was in his fifties, I learned, with advanced lung cancer, and had been receiving hospice care at home over the past three weeks. He was married and had three children and many grandchildren living nearby (this was a relatively small town). He had given no warning to anyone that he planned to take his life. Nor could the hospice staff understand why he did.

What made Michael's suicide particularly confusing to them was that they thought that he could have lived for several months. Moreover, those months probably would have been reasonably good. Michael had no symptoms of pain, or nausea, or shortness of breath. And although it's true that he was often tired, and couldn't be as active as he'd once been, he was still able to take short walks in a nearby park with his beagle, Sam. He could attend parties and occasional dances nearby. Nor was he depressed, as far as anyone knew. In short, there seemed to be no source of physical or emotional suffering that might have motivated him to take his own life. So why did he do it?

I had dinner that night with the hospice medical director, a longtime friend, and a few of the hospice nurses, one of whom had visited Michael and his wife at their home. The conversation was halting at first, as we talked about recent events in the hospice industry and my research project. But Michael's suicide was on everyone's minds, including my own, and the talk soon turned to his death and to his motivations.

I didn't know Michael or his history, so I was silent, listening to the group propose and debate reasons. It was a beautiful night, and we sat around a table on my friend's deck overlooking a small stream. The low, smooth rumble of the water and counterpoint of the crickets in the meadow on the other side made an oddly perfect backdrop for a conversation about what this man had to live for, and what could have motivated him to give that up.

As I listened, they wandered from one explanation to another as an elastic tour group might explore a museum. They would occasionally pause at one explanation before moving on, but would usually circle back, revisiting the same one several times. They drifted separately, for the most part, but sometimes found themselves together for a moment. Finally, close to midnight, they seemed to assemble once more around an explanation that they'd already considered several times.

Michael, they thought, could no longer ignore the telltale signs of his growing dependence on his wife. And he'd begun to place limits on himself and his needs. Too fatigued to be able to shop for himself, for instance, he had begun to make choices about whether to ask his wife to run an errand—for shaving cream, for a magazine, for a fresh bottle of Maker's Mark—or whether to do without. These were little signs, nonevents that we usually don't notice as health care providers. And if we notice them at all, we count these small dependencies as nothing more than the cost of serious illness.

But to Michael these signs meant much more. These requests to his wife were a series of pointillist dots that, viewed together, gave him a picture of the increasing burden that he was placing almost entirely on his wife's shoulders. The group thought that this mean-ing—meaning that was laced with fear of being a burden—was the driving force for Michael's suicide.

I've recounted Michael's story in lectures to medical students or nursing students, and many seem to grasp his situation intuitively. Even if they don't support his choice, they understand it on a vis-ceral level. Perhaps Michael's fear of being a burden resonates so strongly with them because most of them have never, in their adult lives at least, been dependent on others. They've never experienced anything like Michael's state of dependency, and therefore it's par-ticularly terrifying for them.

But more experienced health care providers, and particularly those of us who work in hospice or in geriatrics, see Michael's pre-dicament differently. We've seen our patients cope with diminished functional status and continue to enjoy life, even with a profound degree of dependence. We've seen the processes of negotiation and accommodation that unfold as an illness rearranges both the pa-tient's life and the lives of his or her family. And most important, perhaps, we've come to recognize that, what a patient perceives as a burden of caregiving, family members may see a gift that they're privileged to be able to offer. But to those—like my students, or Mi-chael, or perhaps Jose—without that experience, it is the burdens, and only the burdens, that they see.

This, too, seems to me to be a reason why Jose might have taken his own life. Fiercely independent, he had resisted most of our ef-forts to provide him with additional support at home and to arrange transportation to and from his appointments with us. Indeed, I sus-pect that his loathing of a nursing home was due at least in part to a fear of being wholly dependent on others. I could imagine that for someone like Jose, that fear of being a burden might well have been more frightening than a fear of dying.

Jose

If I'm right, and Jose really did take his own life, each of the motivations I've described seems plausible. They have a salience, and an obviousness, that makes them hard to ignore. And so these were the explanations that took center stage as we all tried to make sense of Jose's death. But there was a piece of the puzzle that we missed.

About a month after Jose died, his landlady called to tell me that his church choir would be holding a special benefit concert to support his favorite local charity. She thought I'd like to know, in case one of our clinic team wanted to go. I was so surprised by this that I don't think I ever properly thanked her for calling me. Instead, I asked about the choir he'd been in. This was a part of Jose's life that I knew nothing about.

Jose hadn't just been "in" a choir, she said proudly. He'd been its director for years. He selected the hymns they sang and did some of the arranging, too. He had led the church's youth choir as well, and he and several of the adult choir members performed at small gatherings in the city, mostly in West Philadelphia.

I didn't know about any of that, she explained, because Jose had stopped singing, oh, at least two years ago. He had lost his voice, she said. Not his actual voice—his speaking voice hadn't changed—but he couldn't sing like he used to be able to. And he had always led the choir with his voice.

So when he lost his voice, he stopped performing, and soon after, he stopped teaching. And when he stepped down as choir director, he quit the choir altogether. That was the beginning of the end for him, she said. I realized then that in all of our discussions about why Jose might have taken his own life, we missed the possibility Jose might have taken his own life simply because his life had lost its meaning.

Actually, aside from sounding trite, that characterization is not quite accurate. We are, all of us, constantly "losing" the meaning that we attach to our lives, as our lives change. The meaning that I attach to everyday events is not what it was a decade ago, or even a year ago. That old meaning has been lost.

But—and this is the important point—it's been replaced by another meaning. I still get up in the morning because I feel I have a compelling reason to do so, although that reason is not the one that motivated me a year ago. And so it's more accurate to say that Jose had not revised his life's meaning to keep pace with his changing circumstances. The result, nevertheless, is the same. Jose must have increasingly found himself without a persuasive, compelling reason to live.

This an important distinction to me, because it suggests that we might have helped Jose to adapt to his changing circumstances. We could have helped him to find a meaning to replace, at least partly, what he had lost when he lost his voice. We could have helped him to create a meaning that would have let him face each day with the confidence of a narrative structure that made sense.

If this sounds hopeless, consider that most of the stories in this book describe, in a sense, people's efforts to recreate a sense of purpose out of changing circumstances. Think about Lacy's attempt to write a book, or Tom's efforts to provide for his family, or even Marie's goal of teaching her family a lesson. They all managed to reconstruct a purpose that gave meaning to lives that had been torn apart and rearranged so viciously by illness. Jack, Lucy, Priscilla, and I might have helped Jose to do this.

This seems obvious to me, but when I try to explain it to medical students, I often meet resistance, at least at first. "Meaning" doesn't appear in most medical textbooks and isn't part of their vocabulary. They're not sure, initially, what it means to say that a life has lost its meaning.

And so I turn to examples that are vivid and dramatic. Examples like that of the twentieth-century French painter Bernard Buffet, who committed suicide when Parkinson's disease had robbed him of his ability to work. Or the Austrian conductor Georg Tintner, who jumped to his death when ill health due to cancer had taken away his ability to lead an orchestra.

Or—a favorite of women medical students—I tell them about Gertrude Bell, who became known as the Queen of Iraq for her accomplishments as an archeologist, diplomat, writer, and spy. Bell was the founder of the Baghdad Archeological Museum, a principal in developing the blueprint for Iraq's independence and, not coincidentally, a close collaborator of the better-known T. E. Lawrence. And so it was from these heights that she fell abruptly when, on a return to England in 1925, she received a diagnosis of what was probably lung cancer. Realizing that this illness would make it impossible to continue the work that she loved, she committed suicide a few months later in Baghdad.

The example that has the greatest impact on my students, though, is not of someone for whom a loss of meaning prompted suicide. Instead, it's an example of someone who fought against that inclination, creating meaning from impossibly bare circumstances. Viktor Frankl is perhaps best known for his work as a psychiatrist, but he was also a Holocaust survivor whose account of that period, *Man's Search for Meaning,* is among the most moving in print. What provides the motive force for Frankl's narrative is faith in the possibility of finding meaning in everyday existence. He is certain, too, that doing so is essential to survival. Without meaning, he said, we lose the will to live.

He was so adamant on this point, perhaps, because he also recognized this danger of treating one's situation as unreal. Those who had begun to regard their existence in the camps as somehow temporary, or "provisional," had taken the first irrevocable steps toward death. The absence of meaning that keeps pace with changing circumstances, he says, results in hopelessness and depression.

Meaning, I think, is what Jose really needed from us. Perhaps not as urgently as he needed pain medication, but it was a need nonetheless. We could have—should have—helped him to reconstruct a sense of meaning that would have given his life the purpose and thus the structure that he was missing when he could no longer sing.

I'm not sure where he could have found that meaning. Maybe in cataloging and finding a home for the thousand-plus gospel records that lined the walls of his apartment. Or maybe in speaking to West Philadelphia youth groups about drug addiction. I don't know what would have been best. But I do know that he needed something, something that would have given him a purpose for staying alive that would have weighed against the fears of a loss of dignity, of dependence, and of placement in a nursing home.

For all of the help that we offered Jose, we did, finally, miss this. In our focus on reducing Jose's fears—about being unable to live independently, about going to a nursing home—we had missed an opportunity to help Jose construct a purpose that he could have balanced against those fears. We tried to alleviate his fear of dying but didn't help him to want to live.

TEN

Christine

Appreciation and Wisdom

Christine

It was my first view of Christine that I remember best—sitting cross-legged on an embroidered cushion, her feet folded beneath her. The fingers of her right hand were stroking Berty, her cat, and the fingers of her left trailed gently on the limestone tiles of her garden patio, as if she were comparing the two textures, appreciating their contrast. With just enough dust to give texture to the air around her, she appeared to be suspended in the dappled light and sliding shadows. For that moment, she seemed to be a part of the garden of lavender, yucca, monkey flower, and white sage around her.

I met Christine on a beautiful January afternoon when I was in San Diego working on a research project—a welcome respite from the East Coast winter. As one of the first steps in that project, I was spending a few days with the intake nurses at San Diego Hospice to try to understand how the hospice enrollment process worked. I wanted to determine how we could study it, so that, ultimately, we could make the process easier for patients and their families.

I was spending the day with Darla, one of the hospice's youngest and most efficient intake nurses. We had already seen three patients, separated by a lurching lunch of chocolate chip cookies as we sailed up Interstate 5 between patients 2 and 3. Darla was hoping that light traffic and a few shortcuts would let her see one more patient before the end of the day.

As we drove across town to Christine's house near the airport, Darla shared what little information she had about her history. She did so partly out of courtesy and partly to make conversation. But also, I think, she was puzzled by Christine's story and wanted a second opinion.

Christine had discovered she was HIV positive about thirteen years ago, Darla told me, an infection she had acquired from her boyfriend at the time. Since then, she had done remarkably well, without complications or medication side effects. But over the last eighteen months or so her infection had become resistant to treatment, with increased viral counts despite numerous changes to her regimen. As if her disease had sensed her new weakness, in the last six months it had produced a profound wasting that had cost Christine 20 percent of her body weight.

Still, Darla was surprised that Christine had chosen to enroll in hospice now, and I agreed that it was odd. Some degree of medication resistance is common in HIV, and is by no means a death sentence. Although the wasting syndrome that accompanies advanced AIDS can be debilitating, it is not in and of itself fatal. Perhaps, I thought, there were other medical issues we didn't know about.

But as Darla told me more, Christine's decision to enroll in hospice seemed even more difficult to explain. For most of the time that she had been HIV positive, Darla said, Christine had been an aggressive advocate for HIV rights. Until recently, in fact, she'd actually been involved in lobbying and protest demonstrations.

As we turned off the highway and descended into a maze of side streets, Darla and I agreed that it was strange to see this firebrand enrolling in hospice. Certainly, Christine didn't sound like someone who would be likely to embrace hospice's notion of a peaceful death. But if she wasn't interested in hospice, then it would be a very short visit. And we'd have time for one more patient today, Darla said happily, reaching for another cookie.

Christine's house was in a cozy middle-class neighborhood. Her street was a mix of ranch homes whose different paint schemes and landscaping disguised—almost—the fact that they were built from a handful of patterns. Christine's house was wholly unexceptional, with white siding and white trim and a neat yard, as if it were hoping to blend in with its neighbors.

Tied with yellow yarn to the handle of the screen door was a handwritten cardboard sign: FOLLOW THE YELLOW BRICK ROAD. Below the text there was a stylized arrow the width of the sign pointing to the right. Like a comic duo, Darla and I looked at each other, then down, then right. Sure enough, there was a gravel path inlaid with clay-fired bricks that had been painted an impossibly bright yellow.

The path proved easy enough to follow, but it wound through a series of twists and turns that seemed designed for no other purpose than to impede our progress. The first loop took us around a stunted but carefully-tended peppermint tree, and the next grazed a fringe of manzanita that left a few petals on Darla's shoulder as she ducked under the lowest branch. As we rounded the house's rear corner, the dense curtain of foliage behind us muffled the sound of children playing in the street and brought us within earshot of a fountain's soft patter. It had taken us no more than half a minute to walk the fifty feet or so from the front door, but the yellow brick road had done its work. Darla's normally driving pace had slowed and we both paused for a moment as we turned the corner to enjoy the scrappy shade of the live oak anchoring the corner of the lot.

Although we were quite close—perhaps fifteen feet away— Christine didn't seem to notice us at first. Almost a part of the garden, she paid no more attention to us than she did to the branch of lavender hanging over her shoulder. She was dark-complexioned, with shoulder-length black hair and black eyes that seemed sunken, peering out over prominent cheekbones. But what I noticed first was the way that her head was tilted back, in a subtle smile, lips slightly open as if she were about to speak. It was an attitude of appreciative response, as if she were listening to the climax of friend's amusing story and was on the verge of laughter.

It was her cat, Berty, who noticed us first. An orange tabby with a pale white face that gave him the look of a miniature lion, he looked up at us as we stood at the edge of the patio. Just as quickly he dismissed us as potential prey, and turned away. But Christine noticed his interest and looked toward us, taking us in without seeming to react. Her gaze was distantly curious, like that of someone who half-watches a television with the sound turned off.

Then she smiled, waved, and Berty leaped off her lap and disappeared into the mock orange behind her. We had broken whatever spell had been in place. But for a moment, at least, I had had a glimpse of the entrancing peacefulness that had become the leitmotif of Christine's life.

When she rose to greet us, the wasting effects of AIDS were obvious. The fingers of her right hand twining around the fringes of her shawl were as slender as the branches of the bougainvillea around us, and her bare feet in sandals had little more color than the limestone tiles beneath them. Yet her voice was surprisingly rich and steady, without a trace of weakness or a hint of defeat. And her smile, quiet and peaceful, didn't seem to belong to the same person who had amassed the pile of medical records that were assembled on the teak table in front of us.

I was delighted when Christine offered us iced tea, with fresh mint from her garden. I couldn't think of anything better. But Darla was focused and efficient—there was still a chance of seeing one more patient today, after all—and she refused. Not wanting to disrupt her routine, I followed her lead, but reluctantly.

So we talked about hospice, or rather Darla talked and Christine and I listened. Surprisingly, after what we'd heard about Christine's past life as an activist, she quickly agreed to enroll. She'd learned everything she could about hospice, she said calmly, and was certain it was the right choice. Darla completed the necessary paperwork, and I helped by reading through the top three medical record folders on the pile, helping Darla to make sure she recorded the correct medications and doses. In less than an hour, we were done.

But there was not enough time then for another patient, and Darla was in no hurry to dive back into San Diego's rush-hour traffic. So as she finished her paperwork, Darla's pace slowed a bit. Christine seemed to sense an opening and offered us iced tea again, tactically offering poppy seed cakes she had just baked. I could see that Darla was weakening but still hesitant, and so I said yes, and Darla gave in.

That, and Berty's return, seemed to change to tone of our visit. The talk turned to Christine's history and, indirectly, to our own. Christine had grown up as an Army brat, spending most of her childhood on bases in Hawaii, including a couple of years off-base near the neighborhood where I'd grown up on the windward coast of Oahu. She had gone to college in San Diego and later, after two years in the Peace Corps in Papua New Guinea, to nursing school. She and Darla, in fact, had been at the same nursing school only a few years apart.

As the air around us cooled and the soft voice of the fountain seemed to become more prominent, we talked about shared memories of people and places. Berty became increasingly restless, sensing, perhaps, that his nocturnal prey were somewhere just beyond the dense border of the foliage that lined the patio. And so Darla and I both got up to leave.

But then Darla did something that surprised me—she asked Christine if she would mind if she came back to visit. This wasn't consistent with the businesslike Darla that I had been shadowing all day, but then again, neither was the past hour we had spent chatting. Christine smiled—of course she was welcome. She looked at me—we were both welcome, anytime.

I said I would love to come back if I didn't have a full day of work at the hospice tomorrow and then a redeye back home that evening. But Christine pointed out that I would have the early evening free. She knew the redeye schedule well from her travels to Washington and New York. She also said that her house was on the way to the airport, and that I should stop by.

And so the following afternoon I threaded my rental car through the same streets that Darla and I had traveled, taking more than a few wrong turns but pulling up, finally, at Christine's house. There was no note this time, so I rang the bell and heard a chime playing a tune—distantly familiar—that I couldn't quite place. Christine met me at the door, dressed much as she had been the previous day, in an expansive silk wrap, this one of a pale blue that seemed to reflect the shadows outside. But she seemed, somehow, more thin and pale than she had been only a day before. Although this apparent transformation was surely no more than a cruel trick of lighting, as she led me into the house I couldn't help thinking that she had crossed an invisible threshold over the course of the afternoon. She seemed, suddenly and inexplicably, like a hospice patient.

Christine led me into the living room, a wide, Saltillo-tiled space that opened out onto the patio. We would need to stay inside for a few minutes, she said. She had bread dough rising and would have to put it in the oven soon.

As we sat down, I noticed that the living room walls were bare of artwork, except for a large corkboard, about 6 by 8 feet, taking up one wall. Scattered across it, in rows and clusters, was an array of maybe a hundred pictures. Some were small, no more than snapshots. Others were larger, including a few 8-by-10s that looked like studio portraits. Several seemed old, and there were even a few small black and white prints scattered among them. Scenes of people—

single and in groups—were mixed with dogs and cats and quite a few touristy shots, including one I thought I recognized as Venice's Accademia Bridge.

Christine saw me looking at the pictures and explained both them and the lack of other artwork. About a year ago, after her HIV had proved to be resistant to multiple drugs, she said, she had begun to think about what was important to her. And she realized how much she valued all the people she had known. She wanted to live with daily reminders around her of those people, and so she had begun to gather pictures of friends, people she had traveled with, and people she'd worked with. So the wall of pictures that began as a small collection over the sideboard in the corner had, gradually, taken over the entire wall.

The doorbell rang again—UPS leaving a package—which reminded me to ask about the melody of the chimes, which I still couldn't quite place. Ponderous, but bouncy. Like a cartoon version of *Pomp and Circumstance.* She laughed—it was "If I Only Had a Brain" from *The Wizard of Oz.*

The yellow brick road, and the door chimes? (And one other clue I had missed). Did she have a *Wizard of Oz* fixation? A Dorothy complex?

No, she laughed. Well, yes, actually. Her Peace Corps days, for instance, were her Dorothy phase. As she flew halfway around the world, she identified with Dorothy's own trip to Oz. At various times of her life, she added, she had identified with other characters, like the Scarecrow (nursing school), and so on.

She explained each one, and they seemed to fit remarkably well. But when she got to the Lion (courage) I had to ask. What had made her—and here I almost said what had made her give up—so peaceful? She wasn't at all the firebrand that I had expected.

She smiled, perhaps because her reputation had preceded her, and probably because she'd heard this question before. She explained that she had been a fighter for quite a while. In fact, for the first five years or so after her diagnosis, she had seen every obstacle—medical and administrative—as a personal affront. When her employer (a hospital) instituted mandatory HIV testing, she saw that policy as a challenge, and, moreover, a challenge that was aimed at her personally. It was her ability to conjure up anger that gave her courage. And it was that anger, then, that guaranteed her a place at the front in a cadre of similar-minded activists who were intent on changing state laws and, later, on taking their battle to Washington.

Her anger and a sense of personal challenge had served as a lifeline of sorts, which she used to haul herself out of a moat of self-pity and despair. Rather than feel sorry for herself, she would get angry. Her activist friends had been through this before, and they saw this transformation as healthy. So they goaded her along, building her anger and discouraging self-pity.

Before long, she said, she came to rely on that anger. She needed it to help her forget her physical illness, and she needed the respite from self-pity that it offered. That anger pulled her out of bed in the morning when she had no energy, and urged her onto a redeye to Washington for a demonstration the next morning when she felt too nauseated to keep anything down.

She also needed her anger in a more fundamental way, Christine told me. It was also her single most reliable link to the activists who were first her supporters and later her compatriots and friends. Anger was the basis of their community and the foundation of her friendships.

But that anger needed to be tended carefully, and without assiduous attention it began to subside. Soon she noticed that it had become unreliable. She would find herself sitting quietly at some meetings. Or she would skip some demonstrations entirely to take a walk and enjoy the sunshine. That made her life unstable. She never knew when she might walk off an edge and lose the anger that had been supporting her.

I had seen a pair of roller skates in a corner of the front hallway. They were the old kind—a tall leather boot on four polyurethane wheels, with a pudgy figurehead of a toe stop—that were meant for skating rinks. And they made me think of Charlie Chaplin's scene in the after-hours department store with Paulette Goddard in *Modern Times*. Blindfolded, he glides in circles and figure eights, forward and backward, all on the store's mezzanine. Again and again he grazes the unprotected edge, each time a little closer, and then—just barely—back to Goddard and safety.

Christine laughed. She knew the scene, and she agreed. But, she pointed out, Chaplin was blindfolded and therefore oblivious. In contrast, she could see the despair and sense of hopelessness beyond the edge. Still, she agreed, for Chaplin's audience, and indeed for her, that experience had been as anxiety-provoking as a horror film.

But she realized that no matter how much she'd come to depend on her activist life and its community, she couldn't sustain those relationships without a stout sense of anger and injustice. So she began to back away from the life she had assembled over the previous ten years. First she stopped attending meetings, where her new passivity was most noticeable. Soon other activities—demonstrations, lobbying visits to Washington—followed.

Her friends were concerned, of course. She herself thought she might be depressed, or perhaps suffering from an early HIV-induced dementia. But her physician reassured her. Besides, Christine said, she didn't feel sad, and she was thinking as clearly as ever, if not more so. She was just . . . peaceful.

That was the point at which, about two years previously, she had begun to spend less time traveling and more time in her garden. As she did, she noticed a stray, underfed tabby and began feeding him, eventually adopting him and naming him Berty. Here Christine gave me a moment's grace period before explaining what I would never have figured out, that "Berty" was in honor of Bert Lahr, who had played the Cowardly Lion.

As she began spending more time at home, there were long periods—hours, sometimes—when she said she felt as if she were sinking into the garden around her. It wasn't meditation, exactly. She'd tried that years before, with limited success. But the sensation was the same sort of selective awareness. In that frame of mind even the smallest events were entrancing. For instance, she described the way the shifting shadows from the live oak would play over a column of ants, making it seem to writhe like a garden snake. Or she would look at the swirls and smudges of dirt and leaves on the limestone tiles, finding patterns inside patterns, like nested Rorschach blots.

Christine seemed more than willing to talk about this, and I was curious. So I asked her why she thought this change happened. And why did it happen when it did?

She had known all along, she told me, that at some point the antiretroviral drugs would not be able to keep pace with her disease. Unlike her activist friends, she couldn't find much comfort in the common wisdom that HIV was just another chronic illness, like diabetes or high blood pressure. People died of diabetes and high blood pressure, didn't they?

So she knew she was living with a death sentence of sorts. She suspected that this knowledge led her to think and feel differently. And she thought it had probably given her, over time, a new appreciation of each day that she felt well.

From there our conversation that evening trailed off in a dozen different directions—growing up in Hawaii, the mechanics of the HIV virus, the politics of AIDS—twining around like the tendrils of bougainvillea. But it was her description of peacefulness that I remember most. It grew dark and an automatic patio light came on, bathing us in a yellow glow that seemed, oddly, like a premature sunrise. I looked at my watch, recalled that I had a rental car to return and a flight to catch, and, finally, got up to leave.

After a hug, and a wave as I rounded the corner of the house, I took a last look back. Christine was seated again on her cushion, the yellow beams of the porch light filtering through the bamboo along the house and playing over her face and Berty's twitching tail as he sat in her lap. Just as she had been the first time Darla and I saw her the day before, Christine seemed composed, peaceful, almost distant, looking up into the now-dark yard with a mixture of peaceful wonder tinged with expectation.

Transformation Near the End of Life

It was that peaceful attitude that I remembered most clearly as I followed the yellow brick road back to my car. And as I drove to the airport and made my way to the gate, I thought about the attitude of acceptance that I had glimpsed that evening. I thought about the transformation that had taken Christine from fire-breathing activism to peaceful acceptance.

She was, I thought, an unusual woman. One who was endowed with far more depth and insight than most people have. One who was able to leave behind the vicissitudes of a devastating chronic illness and who seemed to become another person entirely. That is, I thought of Christine's transformation as the next stage in the development of a remarkable person.

What I didn't consider, at least not initially, was the possibility that the extraordinary person I had just left, and her unique attitude toward life, was to some degree the product of her illness. My vision was restricted by what psychologists call "attribution bias." When we try to explain others' behavior we tend to underestimate the importance of circumstances, placing more emphasis on personality traits. For instance, I interpreted Darla's hard-driving schedule as the product of her youth and energy—her personality—rather than what was, perhaps, simply a busy day.

Similarly, I'd interpreted Christine's peaceful acceptance as the natural and logical result of who she was, rather than as a result of living with a chronic serious illness. She had been influenced by her experiences with HIV, of course. But I discounted those experiences as a potential explanation of the person she'd become. Although I could see that the circumstances of living with HIV might have prompted the sort of transformation that Christine had undergone, I assumed that it was Christine's own unique attributes that made that transformation possible.

But on the turbulent and therefore sleepless flight home that night, I began to look at her transformation differently. Christine was certainly unique, and special. Distance hadn't altered my thinking about her qualities. Still, somewhere over the wheat fields of South Dakota, I began to wonder whether her knowledge that death was close, albeit still uncertain, might have been a goad to developing the sort of peaceful appreciation that she had discovered.

I realized, of course, that this was hardly an original notion. In fact, there is a widespread expectation that proximity to death brings some sort of positive transformation along the lines of what Christine seemed to have experienced. No less an authority than the Bible tells us that if we recognize that our lives are finite, we become wiser. "So teach us to number our days, that we may apply our hearts unto wisdom." (Psalm 90:12; King James Version). Other translations make this link even more clear by promising, for instance, that by numbering our days we "may learn wisdom" (Revised English Bible).

Nevertheless, it's taken me far more time than my flight home that night afforded to understand how I felt about the possibility that Christine was at least in part the product of her circumstances. On one hand, it was an uncomfortable rearrangement. I was surprised and a bit unnerved by the possibility that at least some of what I had witnessed was not a reflection of who Christine was, but was instead the product of her circumstances. It was, I thought, a little like Dorothy's realization that the Wizard was not so great and powerful after all.

On the other hand, this view of Christine's transformation was strangely attractive. The idea that proximity to death can be transformative—for anyone—has democratic, egalitarian implications that I find very appealing. It's reassuring to think that this opportunity for transformation is available to everyone in her circumstances.

And it's reassuring, too, to think that the experience of facing death can bring with it the strength to meet that experience. This equation reminds me of something my more devoutly religious patients tell me, that God doesn't give them misfortunes that He doesn't think they will be able to manage. They find this notion comforting because it links their suffering to their strength. It reassures them that whatever misfortune befalls them won't overwhelm them. In the same way, I'd like to think that while Christine's experience with a serious illness challenged her, it also gave her the worldview and attitude to meet that challenge.

The Transformation Process

I know that I'm not alone in finding comfort in the notion that serious illness can confer a sense of peace and acceptance. Not only is this hopeful idea woven into cultural references as far back as the Bible, but it's also a central element of much of the earliest research related to death and dying. For instance, Elisabeth Kübler-Ross's stages of dying constitute a path that leads to some form of acceptance and, presumably, the sense of peace that acceptance brings. Indeed, this promise was probably responsible in large part for her theory's popularity.

One of the earliest accounts of the transformative power of approaching death comes not from a psychologist or a physician but, strangely, from a geologist. Albert von St. Gallen Heim was a distinguished professor at the University of Zurich in the late nineteenth and early twentieth centuries who became fascinated—obsessed, really—with documenting the phenomenology of the near-death experience. As an avid climber, Heim had had several close encounters with death himself. These episodes, together with others that he witnessed or heard about, led him to wonder whether there are patterns of experience under those circumstances.

So over the course of several years he collected stories of people who narrowly escaped death in falls from bridges, ice shelves, and alpine crags. The centerpiece of this collection, not surprisingly, was a detailed account of his own near-deadly fall of some 70 feet in 1871. He sums up his own experience and the experiences of others with enviable confidence. "In nearly 95% of the victims," he concludes, "there occurred, independent of the degree of their education, thoroughly similar phenomena, experienced with only slight differences."

Although he is describing actual events in the past, Heim has an odd predilection to discuss them in the future tense, as if his chief goal is to reassure readers that these experiences are not so bad. The victim's sense of time will slow down, he promises, becoming "greatly expanded." He also remarks on an enhanced mental activity and sense of clarity that the experience seems to confer. You will feel a "calm seriousness," he predicts, and a sense of "profound acceptance." You will be unworried, yet with the "dominant mental quickness and sense of surety" to save yourself if survival is possible. And, perhaps inevitably, the victim often hears beautiful music as he falls through "a superbly blue heaven containing roseate cloudlets." Reading Heim's promises of peace, calm, music and beauty is hypnotic.

Indeed, his paper reads in many places like the bland reassurance of a competent anesthesiologist describing an upcoming surgical procedure. There will be no anxiety, no grief or despair, Heim claims. Nor will there be any pain. Heim is particularly clear about this point, emphasizing it several times throughout the paper. "A scream," Heim reports, in a not-particularly-convincing effort to be reassuring, "was hardly ever heard." In the end, it is the absence of suffering that I find so appealing in Heim's account. And this is, probably, precisely what Heim intended.

It would be nice to know, with the same certainty that Heim

seems to enjoy, that our deaths due to other causes will follow a similar pattern. I'd like to be certain, for instance, that all of us will experience the same sense of peaceful acceptance and appreciation that a climber experiences as he falls toward an inhospitable slab of rock at a predetermined terminal velocity of—I'm told—about 125 miles per hour. I'd like very much to believe that Heim's generalizations are true, and that they hold as well for people with terminal illness.

But they don't. I've cared for only a few patients who were transformed as completely as Christina was. On the other hand, I've cared for many more who found some fraction of the peace and tranquility that Christine discovered. Still, the path that Christine took in the last year or two of her life was both remarkable and, I think, unique.

In fact, the notion that we will all undergo some sort of thorough transformation can create unrealistic expectations. For instance, when I think about any of my patients in terms of Kübler-Ross's stages, it's hard not to think in terms of their progress, or lack thereof. Any model of transformation that includes discrete stages, whether it's those of Kübler-Ross or the transformation that Heim described, asks us to place people in categories, distinguishing them by how close they have come, or not, to a goal.

These expectations can be troubling. I took care of a very young patient once who had just been diagnosed with a particularly rare and deadly form of leukemia. The best prognosis was that aggressive treatment would help him to live for another two years. A cure, in his case, wasn't possible. He was a college student and had read *On Death and Dying* for a class, never imagining any more than any of us would, that its lessons would apply to him. And so he asked the medical student who was assigned to him when he could expect to feel better. Could he expect to reach the stage of acceptance by the time he was discharged from the hospital?

As health care providers, we are all at risk of falling into the trap that claimed that patient. Like Heim, most of us want to believe in the potential of a sudden, dramatic transformation. There is something optimistic about the possibility that peace and acceptance lie waiting for us after some significant event or development, or perhaps simply when we wake up tomorrow morning. All science aside, it's comforting to know that a mental transformation is possible.

Moreover, we tell ourselves, we've seen these cases. These are the patients like Christine, whom we remember clearly. More than that, these are the cases that we bring out and share with each other. Like proud parents carrying their children's pictures within quick-draw reach, we take these examples out and pass them around. Their simplicity is mysterious—almost magical—and therefore, somehow inspiring.

Although I'd like very much to believe that all of my patients could experience the sort of transformation that Christine did, with the suddenness that Heim's accounts promise, I recognize that reality is much more complicated. Kübler-Ross's stages offer an enticing conceptual model, but it's a model that doesn't really predict the experience of most patients. And this tension between a simple and appealing theory of stages, on one hand, and a more complex reality of gradual change, on the other, has an antecedent in an earlier debate about—of all things—evolution.

In the nineteenth century there were two competing theories of evolution: one described the process of speciation as happening in sudden leaps; the other posited gradual and almost imperceptible steps. Scholars of that period were attracted by the simple elegance of sudden speciation. At the same time, though, they were forced to acknowledge substantial evidence to the contrary. Their predicament was, I think, not unlike the way that I find myself torn between two visions of the transformation process near the end of life.

In an effort to bridge the gap between the two theories, Richard Goldschmidt, a German-born geneticist, suggested that the development of new traits was gradual, as individuals accrued a series of mutations. At some point those mutations fused together to form what was immediately recognizable as a new species. In a burst of poetic license that was probably partly responsible for his theory's demise (its lack of scientific justification played a significant role as well), Goldschmidt coined the term "hopeful monsters" to describe those individuals in which invisible mutations were accruing.

Sadly, just as his theory has been discredited in favor of a more pedestrian, gradualist understanding of evolution and speciation, much the same has happened, for better or worse, with stage theories of dying. "Sadly," to me at least, because I love the idea implicit in Goldschmidt's theory that there may be transformative changes happening, quietly and invisibly, beneath the surface. Changes that I and perhaps not even my patients are aware of. It's reassuring for me to think that my patients might actually be carrying, unknowingly, almost all of the elements of such a transformation. They're just waiting for some event, some trigger, to make the transformation complete.

I also like Goldschmidt's theory because it reminds me that transformative changes might be occurring independently of anything my colleagues and I do or say. I've become humbled over time by the limits that circumscribe what health care providers can accomplish, and the assistance that physicians in particular can provide. Indeed, most of the transformation and growth that patients can expect will happen without my help. It's comforting, therefore, to think that some of my patients at least are playing host to these sorts of changes, unbeknownst to them, and independent of anything I could do.

Themes of Transformation

If you accept, as I've come to, that some sort of transformation is possible, even usual, what might that transformation look like? Are there ways of living and looking at the world and ourselves that recur? Perhaps not with the rigid universality that Heim imagined, but at least with some consistency across diverse circumstances and settings?

In fact, there are two overlapping themes that I've seen many times. One is that my patients seem to perceive time differently. A second—linked, perhaps, to the first—is that my patients often develop a new appreciation for things that they had previously taken for granted. When these changes happen, they seem to me to be ingredients of other, more far-reaching changes in priorities, lifestyles, and relationships, and they can explain many of the other changes that my patients undergo.

First, many of my patients tell me they experience an altered perception of time. Not coincidentally, this is a prominent feature of the accounts that Heim collected as well. Although this rearrangement of time is likely to be most extreme, and most obvious, in the dramatic events that Heim describes, it occurs in some form among my patients with serious illnesses. Christine, for instance, told me vividly about how she could become immersed in a single moment that would become drawn out over hours. She described, too, the sensation of time disappearing and leaving her living, purely, in the present.

Consider for a moment the thoughts that occupy you every day. Many of them touch on the future. Next summer's vacation, for instance, or a child's graduation from college, or your eventual retirement. Now imagine being faced with an illness that will end your life in several months. Imagine editing those thoughts constantly, even obsessively, to eliminate those that include a future that is now unreachable—skipping over musings about a child's career choice, for instance, or cutting short daydreams about a retirement plan that is no longer relevant.

This editing naturally foreshortens the scope of time that seriously ill patients have in front of them. No longer thinking in terms of decades or even years, my patients have to force themselves to focus instead much more narrowly. Closing doors that lead to the distant future, they inhabit a temporal corridor that includes only the next few weeks.

This sense of finite time, of a lifetime that is shrinking day by day, conspires to enhance our perceptions of the world around us. It forces us to pay attention, to see, and to appreciate things that we hadn't noticed before. That was certainly true for Christine, who had an enthusiasm not unlike that of the classic Epicurean notion of a quiet, "static" sort of pleasure. The pleasure, for instance, of reminiscence, as in the pictures that lined the corkboard on one wall. Or the smell of fresh-baked muffins. Or the feel of the sunlight brushed rhythmically back and forth by the leaves of the live oak that stretched above her.

Those moments of quiet enjoyment—appreciation, really— remind me of a moment that Viktor Frankl describes: a cattle car full of men being transported to Auschwitz, clutching at a glimpse of the Bavarian Alps around Salzburg. He seems surprised, and a little bit relieved, that these men could appreciate the beauty that they saw framed by the bars of their prison on wheels. Despite the fact that they were being deported to their deaths, or perhaps precisely because of that fact, Frankl says, they were "carried away by nature's beauty." It's remarkable to me, though, how often these moments of appreciation are hidden behind more salient motivations and goals. In fact, these moments tend to disappear from view entirely, unless they're noted and recorded by someone who is perceptive enough to recognize their value. They play a very small part, for instance, in Harold Brodkey's remarkable, and remarkably dense, memoir *This Wild Darkness*. And yet these moments are what I remember best from his account of his last year of life.

When I think about the year he describes, his truculent battles with his physician are vague, smudged like a charcoal sketch by time and wear. Other moments, though, are still as bright and luminous in my mind as some of the most moving Dutch masters' scenes. And indeed they have much the same content, that of quiet everyday scenes that easily slip by unnoticed. The summer afternoon he spent reading quietly with his wife, Ellen, on the porch of their summer house, or a dinner with friends on the Grand Canal in Venice, or watching Ellen tend their garden. Even tinged with sadness—as he realized he was becoming too weak to read or travel, and that their garden was now her garden—these were the moments that seemed to me to pull Brodkey from one moment to the next. And it was scenes like these that Brodkey captured so perfectly because, I think, he lived them so thoroughly.

The quiet enjoyment that Christine and Brodkey and Frankl experienced remind me of a woman I met once in Iowa for whom sunrises had become an almost religious ritual of appreciation. After a night on call at the university hospital, when I found myself awake early, I'd get a cup of coffee from one of the nurses' stations and climb the stairs to a bridge connecting two buildings on the seventh floor. Little more than a hallway, it offered unparalleled views of the surrounding countryside. All the way to Missouri, or Minnesota, I told myself. Or to the Mississippi River to the east.

There was something magical about a sunrise seen from that hallway after a night on call spent saving lives, or trying to, at least. Looking out over the sleeping town of Iowa City and the farms stretching off toward the horizon, I could easily entertain a sort of Holden Caulfield–like delusion that I was somehow a protector, a savior. Mostly, though, I came for the view.

And the view was magnificent, particularly in the winter. In partial recompense, I suppose, for the bone-squeezing cold of its harsh winter, Iowa sunrises in January and February were stunning. The ultimate black of an Iowa night would begin to dissolve, growing more blue and—if possible—even colder. Then a warm glow of light would come rolling across the endless flat fields to the east, seeming to warm everything in its path as it raced toward me. It was always worth the trip, and worth the sacrifice of a few minutes that I should have used to check labs or write orders. An added appeal for me was that I almost always found myself alone, a welcome respite from the pressure of twenty-four hours of calls to answer and problems to solve.

But one morning in January, I walked out onto the bridge to find that a patient had arrived before me. Alone, Lana was sitting in a wheelchair. She was impossibly thin and pale, with almost translucent skin. Even 20 feet away, I could see the thin blue veins in one hand as it hung at her side. She was wearing a respiratory isolation mask and I guessed—correctly, as it turned out—that she was a patient on the leukemia unit, next door to the oncology ward where I was working that month. She seemed so depleted that I thought at first that she had walked here by herself, pushing the chair in front of her, and was simply stopping to rest. But she was turned to face the east, in much the same position that I usually took up, between two pillars that flanked one of the largest windows. I realized that she was there for the same reason that I was.

We watched that sunrise together, silently, for what was perhaps five minutes. As I sipped acrid nurses'-station coffee, she sat there, still and unmoving. And then, just as I was turning to leave, Lana began clapping softly. She wasn't looking at me, and in fact she hadn't given any indication that she noticed I was there. Her applause seemed like a spontaneous and unselfconscious form of appreciation.

I was on call again four nights later, and the next morning I was on the bridge again. And again Lana had arrived there before me. There was a cloud bank far to the east over the Mississippi River, the last trace of a storm that had quietly left 6 inches of snow on the ground the night before. That show was less dramatic, more subtle. A connoisseur's sunrise. No flash of light but, in its place, a gradual warming of the sky and snow-covered fields that slid across the spectrum from deep black through a cobalt blue to a splendid yellow-orange.

Again she clapped in appreciation. More slowly, I thought, but with a determined sort of enthusiasm. She must have known that I was there, yet she didn't turn to acknowledge me. Nor did she give any indication that her applause had an audience, although again I felt as though her rhythmic clapping was intended at least partly for me. In fact, I'd begun to interpret her applause as a gentle reprimand. As a reminder that one shouldn't walk away from such a show without offering some sort of acknowledgment.

I was tempted to imitate her, but I didn't. It seemed too theatrical, too forced. As soon as I pushed open the heavy fire door at one end of the bridge, though, I regretted not joining her. The hospital was a community of transients, I knew. Whoever she was, she would probably be discharged before I was on call next.

And so I was surprised to see Lana again, four mornings later. But this time there was someone with her. An older woman—her mother, perhaps—noticed me and offered a nod and a smile that were friendly and, I thought, a little conspiratorial.

The sky had clouded over during the previous night, bringing sleet and ice. The light that filtered through revealed a solid metallic sheet of clouds stretching to the horizon. For a moment, though, the sun found its way through the narrow gap just below the clouds, illuminating a distant stretch of farmland ahead of the front's leading edge. Neither grand nor impressive, it was a little like a glimpse of a stage from the very back row of a grand auditorium. It was a scene, I thought, that demanded the work of imagination.

But Lana must have decided that this was as good as it was going to get. And so she began to clap in the same measured cadence that she had used before. Her mother looked at me quickly with a half-smile that seemed intended as a tolerant apology, as if she were embarrassed by her daughter's behavior.

Feeling guilty for the previous mornings on which I'd walked away quietly, this time I joined her. A bit too enthusiastically. Enthusiastically enough, anyway, to startle her mother, who looked at her daughter and at me as if she had stumbled across some strange pagan ritual. In a sense, I suppose she had.

On the two previous mornings I had left first, pulled away by work that was waiting for me. But this time Lana's mother—impatient with an agenda of her own—turned the chair to leave, and I ended up walking behind the two of them. Suspecting that we were both going to the oncology wards, I offered to push the wheelchair. Up close, I realized that Lana couldn't have been more than twenty-five or so. Her hair—thinned by chemotherapy—made her seem much older, although up close she seemed, if anything, more frail and vulnerable, taking up barely half of the chair's narrow seat.

Lana was silent on the elevator ride down as her mother, warming to the idea of a doctor escorting her daughter, prattled away. She tired, soon, of the obvious topic of conversation—the sunrise we had just witnessed—and moved on. With a parent-caregiver's sure-footedness in making conversation in uncomfortable situations, she slid easily to the other obvious topic, that of her daughter and a young doctor without a wedding ring. She had no idea, when she had offered to push her daughter upstairs that morning, that she would be meeting someone. Such a handsome and eligible young doctor. And she rambled on, keeping up a steady flow of chatter as if that were her job.

This line of conversation, which would have been awkward enough under the best of circumstances, became acutely uncomfortable as I realized who Lana was. I had never met her but she had been "signed out" to me every night I had been on call. Only nineteen years old, she'd been diagnosed with a smooth muscle tumor that had grown aggressively throughout her back, causing significant pain and paralysis. (I realized then that she had probably never propelled her own wheelchair up to the bridge, as I had assumed. She had been brought there, presumably, by a nurse's aide. And I'd left her there as I hurried back to my work.)

Lana was visibly annoyed, at first, by the line that her mother's conversation was taking. But she caught my eye as I turned her wheelchair around in the elevator. I smiled—fuel for her mother's fire, had she been paying attention—and Lana relaxed as she saw that I was used to this sort of thing.

When we arrived at the oncology ward, her mother left us alone to make a phone call, or so she claimed. Lana was apologetic. Her mother was disappointed, she said, that all of the doctors on her ward were women or married men. I was the first eligible bachelor her mother had seen and she was overreacting.

But, she was quick to say, she wasn't really in a dating mood. I said that was all right; I hadn't really been stalking her, despite the way that it might have seemed. I told her how I loved to watch the sunrise after a night on call.

That's when she told me a little about her own sunrises. She had always liked that moment of the day best, she said. Hopefulness about a new day, tinged with pride at being awake before anyone else. Quiet, too. She enjoyed the quiet, particularly on a winter morning.

But more than anything, Lana said, she knew that she didn't have too many sunrises to look forward to. I didn't protest, although in any other setting etiquette would have demanded it. I knew enough about her medical condition to know that she was probably right. And I think she would have been surprised, and maybe hurt, if I had doled out the same empty reassurance that I imagine she got from her mother. It was true that she didn't have too many sunrises left, and she was right to want to enjoy every one.

And, she said, the funny thing was that she did enjoy every one. Each one, honestly, a little more than the last. Lana said this as if she couldn't quite believe it. Or as if she didn't think I would believe it, or perhaps both. But she repeated it, as if trying to convince both of us. That these sunrises just keep getting more beautiful. And she could hardly wait to see what the next one would be like. She was grateful for that, she said.

What I remember best from that exchange was not only her sense of appreciation, but a corresponding sense of gratitude. Gratitude that she had the chance to see one more sunrise. And gratitude that the last one was as beautiful as it was. That explained her ritual-istic applause every morning, I think. It was her way of giving thanks.

As it turned out, Lana had only a few sunrises left. The next night I was on call her intern told me that she had developed kidney failure due, probably, to the tumor having wrapped around her kid-neys, blocking them entirely. She and her parents had decided not to try to bypass the obstruction surgically. Doing so would just be a temporary measure anyway. She had lost consciousness, he said, and would probably die that night or the following day.

The next morning the sunrise wasn't particularly spectacular. It was abrupt and unsentimental. Night then day. Nothing special. At least, that's what I would have told her, but she wouldn't have be-lieved me.

Wisdom

What I noticed first about Christine, and the image that I carried with me on the flight home, was a peacefulness that was so at odds with the way that she had been while she was healthy. I saw her ability to live in the moment, for instance, and her appreciation of simple things like freshly baked bread and a quiet afternoon with Berty in her garden. I saw all this clearly. And I congratulated myself, I suppose, for being perceptive enough to notice it.

What I didn't notice until much later was that Christine had also developed new priorities. And that she'd also shifted the way in which she balanced those priorities. The result—which I didn't really appreciate at the time—was a transformation in the way that she spent her time.

She'd forsaken politics and advocacy in favor of time with friends, for instance. She'd begun to avoid travel whereas in the past she'd sought out opportunities for adventure. And she was learning to seek enjoyment and satisfaction in small, simple pleasures rather than in grand projects and ideas. Christine, I think, had discovered a form of wisdom. That is, she'd found a way to make the "right"—for her—choices about how to spend her time. This is perhaps a simplistic definition of wisdom, yet it is not too different from Aristotle's view of practical wisdom, or *phronesis*. Someone with practical wisdom, he says, is someone who can "deliberate well." This is more or less what Christine did when she took stock of her options and chose to leave politics and advocacy for a simpler, more peaceful life.

If wisdom is "deliberating well," then it seems to me that wisdom, or something very much like it, can be inspired by life-threatening illness. Indeed, I think that many of the patients that I've described in other chapters were given a similar opportunity to deliberate well. Some of these rose to the challenge. Ladislaw, for instance, found a purpose and pursued it with an enviable clarity and confidence. Alberto recognized, just in time, that his family was more important than concealing his past. Marie found a creative compromise between her love for her family and her equally strong desire to teach them a lesson.

For others, though, wisdom didn't seem to arrive in time. Jerry, for instance, couldn't see past his own view of his illness and morality to recognize that others needed an apology from him. Or Jose, who saw clearly all that he had lost, but who couldn't imagine the meaning that he might still create from the days he had left.

But even for those like Jerry or Jose who seem to go astray, there is sometimes time for wisdom to appear at the last moment. My favorite example of this comes from *Ikiru*, the 1952 Akira Kurosawa film about a bureaucrat diagnosed with advanced cancer whose first response is to repair to a bar to drink and forget. But that initial night of drinking leads to a gradual awakening and a recognition of what was important to him—building a playground in a poor section of town. In the end, he is remembered in the community not as a bureaucrat but as someone to be emulated.

It may be incorrect, however, to say that the proximity to death confers wisdom. Indeed, death need not be a certainty, or even a high probability, in order to rearrange our priorities. Many of my patients, for instance, continue to imagine death as probable, or merely possible, up until their final hours. Nevertheless, they rearrange their lives and priorities, acting as if they were going to die soon. And the reverse is true as well, of course. There are those, like Jacob, who knew with utter certainty that he was going to die, yet didn't rearrange his priorities at all.

So wisdom seems to require, above all, a sort of fearless imagination. An ability to imagine death as a possibility, for instance. And, moreover, a willingness to engage that possibility and to think seriously about what one might do differently.

Therefore, it's probably more accurate to say that any newfound wisdom in a setting of serious illness is the product of living with the possibility of death. In fact, there is evidence that living with chronic illness—even without the possibility of death—does lead to a rearrangement of goals and priorities. Such rearrangements are so well described, in so many settings, that they seem to have a biological basis.

As we experience pleasure or pain, our impressions of those stimuli undergo a variety of changes that are known collectively as "adaptation." Because we experience an event in reference to the events that preceded it, as our situation improves or, in the case of chronic illness, becomes worse, these trends will influence the way that we perceive the next event. The result is that, as chronic illness progresses, our expectations of what it means to be happy, functional, and fulfilled change. We may lose the ability to drive, or to climb stairs, or even to walk. These are deficits that, to a healthy person at least, seem to be devastating. They are the sorts of deficits that healthy people say would make their lives no longer worth living. And yet, when you ask people with these deficits, and even those with deficits that are much more severe, they often say that life is not so bad. They have adapted to their limitations and circumstances.

Of all the studies of adaptation, the most convincing by far involve accident victims who have suffered serious spinal cord injuries and are left with paralysis from the neck down (quadriplegia) or from the waist down (paraplegia). These are people who suddenly found themselves unable to do virtually anything that they had done only days before. This is the sort of situation—a sort of accelerated version of chronic illness, in which losses accumulate rapidly—that should lead people to give up. At the very least one would think that people who had endured such a dramatic change would conclude that life is no longer worth living.

And some do, at least in the first days and weeks after their accident. But as time passes, people with these sorts of injuries express levels of satisfaction with their lives not so different from those of similar people who were not injured. That is, they seem to find a new "set point" that allows for happiness, contentment, and fulfillment under what appear to be vastly reduced circumstances.

To some extent, of course, this adaptation is simply the result of reduced expectations and perhaps a new frame of reference. For instance, a person with paraplegia may be grateful that he still has most or all of his upper body strength. But it's also likely, I think, that many of those who suffer losses of function find alternative sources of satisfaction. Some go back to school, or find fulfillment in other activities that don't require physical function.

Their stories may be extreme, but they are hardly unusual. Most if not all of my patients who live with chronic serious illness are forced to give up at least some of what makes life meaningful for them. But many find alternatives. One of my favorite examples is that of a long-haul trucker I took care of once who had lost his driver's license years earlier to Parkinson's disease. No longer able to drive at all, he still loved watching the countryside unfold in front of him. And so he developed a fascination with trains, taking long trips up and down the East Coast and, once, across the country. It was all for the best, he told me. If he hadn't lost his license, he never would have discovered how wonderful it could be to take a train all the way to Los Angeles. His expectations had shifted, but so, too, had his priorities.

Of course, there is reason to be skeptical that serious illness and the possibility of death bring wisdom. For instance, I'll admit that some of what I'm calling "wisdom" is actually an interpretation that we impose on our choices. By dressing those choices in a costume of wisdom, and by telling ourselves that the circumstance of facing death helps us to make better choices, we may simply be convincing ourselves that our choices are the best. That is, if approaching death brings wisdom, then the choices we're making must necessarily be the right ones. Still, so many of the choices that my patients make seem clearly to be the right ones—"right" for them—that I really do think that there is a strong case for the possibility of wisdom emerging near the end of life.

Christine

I wonder what Christine would have said if I had described this theory to her as we sat talking in her garden? Would she have agreed with the notion that her illness gave her a different perception of time? Or with the idea that a different perception of time led her to a greater appreciation of things that she had previously taken for granted? And what about my suggestion that her illness and changing perceptions led her to something resembling wisdom?

She might have listened patiently to theories of time and appreciation, but the idea of wisdom, I think, would have amused her. She was quick to laugh at herself, and she was modest about her own accomplishments. I can't imagine her admitting to anything like wisdom, even if that wisdom was brought by her illness. So although I wonder what Christine would have thought about all of these theories, perhaps it's just as well that I didn't ask.

Besides, I prefer the idealized image that I have of her, undiluted by modesty. That image is of someone who recognized the limits of the time that she had left and who began to appreciate, in a quiet way, the beauty around her. And, finally, it's an image of someone for whom those fundamental rearrangements led her to adjust her priorities, making her wiser in the process. That's the image I carry forward as I think about how she might have spent the last months of her life.

She had reached, I thought, a sort of equilibrium with her illness. It was what engineers (and Wallace Stegner, in his novel of this title) refer to as an "angle of repose." The term refers to the angle of a hillside that is shallow enough that sand, gravel, and boulders come, finally, to rest. It's the point at which friction fights to a stalemate with gravity, and all motion stops. And that's how I like to think of Christine when I met her, as having reached, finally, a stable equilibrium, an angle of repose.

And so I'm glad, in a way, that I don't know much about what her final months were really like. I have some idea. I know, for instance, that the last time I heard from Darla, about two months later, Christine was still alive and living at home, but she needed increasing help around the house. No longer able to get around easily, she was also beginning to show signs of cognitive impairment. She was relying increasingly on friends and neighbors. Soon, Darla thought, she would need to move to a nursing home.

So Christine's circumstances were changing, and she had not reached the stable equilibrium that I had convinced myself I had seen. I wonder whether she would have been able to maintain the same peaceful appreciation as her home was increasingly overrun by friends and neighbors? And, later, by professional help—nurses and nurse's aides? And would her attitude have withstood a move to a nursing home?

Perhaps I'm not giving Christine enough credit. Just as I had assumed at first that whatever transformation she had undergone was the product of her personality and who she was, perhaps I'm making the same mistake now. Perhaps the changes in her future would motivate rearrangements in Christine's view of the world, and her priorities would shift, just as they had in the past.

I prefer to remember her as I saw her for the first and last time, sitting in her garden, with Berty, surrounded by carefully selected reminders that her life was as she wanted it to be. Pictures of friends on the walls, Berty in her lap, and poppy seed muffins in the oven. And, perhaps, visitors and interesting conversation to look forward to.

Conclusion

The process of writing this book has been challenging, enlightening, and enjoyable in equal measure. But it's been uncomfortable, too, because of the reflection that it's demanded. In trying to recall the details of these stories, I've watched each one scroll by again and again, each time catching a glimpse of another question I should have asked and another clue that, perhaps, I should have noticed. In particular, Sylvester's question to me that night several years ago is one that I've seen more times than I can count. And each time I review that conversation, I wonder what I could have said, or what I could have asked.

This sense of reliving missed opportunities is an uncomfortable feeling, but it's one that's also strangely familiar. In most of my research studies I use open-ended questions whenever I can, because they allow patients and families considerable latitude in the answers that they give. In effect, open-ended questions let them reframe our research questions in a way that makes sense to them. But these questions tend to create unpredictable conversations—the product of a complex interaction between the interviewer, the patient, and his or her family—that move in surprising directions. So rather than trying to herd the dialogue toward a goal that I have in mind, I usually let it find its own path. The interviewers record the resulting conversations so that we can listen to them later and, we hope, piece together a story that makes sense.

Those listening sessions are both fascinating and frustrating. Fascinating, because of what they teach us, but frustrating, too, because for every question that we wrote into our script, our patients' and families' answers suggested many more questions that we didn't think to ask.

In a typical session, my research assistants and I listen to recordings of one or two interviews. More, sometimes, if the interviews were short. We usually sit huddled around a scuffed conference table in my office, leaning close to the tape recorder like a family of the twenties around a radio, sifting through the static to hear muffled voices. We listen, first, to one of my research assistants asking a scripted question. Then we listen to the patient's response. And then—the worst part—we all think of the follow-up question we hope the research assistant asked. This is the question that would help us understand the first answer, usually. Or it's a question that would expand that answer, keeping the conversation going.

Sometimes that question is asked, perhaps even more clearly than we had hoped. When that happens, we heave a collective sigh of relief. But sometimes—not often, but often enough—there is no follow-up question. The interview moves on, and the tape keeps rolling, and we all realize the opportunity that we missed.

The process of writing this book has given me much the same feeling. In fact, it often feels like what strings these disparate stories together are my mistakes. On a bad day, I remember the patients I've described as a series of missed opportunities. They're reminders of questions I should have asked, and occasionally advice I should have offered.

A very wise physician who was a mentor to me as a medical student, Eugene Hirsch, once warned me that leaving mistakes behind is one of the most essential skills of a physician. Review them, of course, and learn from them if you can, he said. But then leave them behind you. Because over the course of a lifetime even the most skilled physician will amass too great a collection of mistakes to carry. In writing this book I've been pleasantly surprised to find that I've managed to let many of these mistakes go. Even those that I still find myself carrying don't seem to have the same weight that they used to.

And I've been no less surprised to find that I've also learned from these mistakes. I've come to understand, for instance, why I was totally unable to answer Sylvester's question to me that night. His question—what should he do with the time he had left?—was one I hadn't heard before. So there was an element of surprise that left me befuddled.

But there was, too, a sort of ponderous urgency to his question that was intimidating. Sylvester had no more than a month or two before he died, if he was lucky. And there was nothing about his medical history that could possibly be described as "lucky." So I recognized that any suggestions I offered would have to be implemented quickly. We'd need to organize and orchestrate, rapidly coordinating the elements of whatever plan we agreed on. It would be a race, I thought.

That sense of urgency provoked in me a profound anxiety about doing, or saying, the wrong thing. I was afraid of being responsible for a word or phrase—perhaps uttered as a casual aside—that would send Sylvester tearing after an impossible goal. Or worse, after a goal that was achievable but ill advised.

And if I've begun to understand why Sylvester's question to me that evening was so difficult, I've also realized that, somewhere in the years that have passed since then, it's become easier to answer. Indeed, it's become something of a welcome challenge. Now when I listen to patients' stories—their medical history, symptoms, and goals for care—I find myself looking for ways to introduce Sylvester's question into our conversations. I've become comfortable enough with the discussions it provokes that I don't even wait until my patients ask me. I find I'm much more willing to start these conversations myself, if I sense a patient is ready.

Why this newfound assurance with a topic that, not too long ago, sent me scrambling to safety? There are, I think, two interwoven answers. First, I've retreated from the rather grandiose role of an advisor—an expert—that I assumed Sylvester wanted me to play. That had been my role throughout our conversation, and I willingly provided the information and advice that he wanted. But his final question to me didn't need an answer. Instead, if he needed anything from me, he only needed me to ask the right questions. This, then, is what I realized I could offer my patients. Not specific guidance about what to do, or what not to do. But questions that might help them to stumble on the right answers on their own.

So what are the right questions? Here, too, I find myself strangely reluctant to make sweeping pronouncements. Still, there are two general guides. These are, in a sense, the broadest possible formulations of the questions that I wish that I had asked Sylvester.

Who, Not What

The question that Sylvester asked me was what he should do with the remaining month or two that he would have before he died. It's a question whose blunt directness mirrored Sylvester's own style, and it's one that goes straight to the heart of the matter. But I've begun to think that a better question to ask, or at least one that would be more useful for most of us, is more oblique.

Perhaps a better question is not what is most important, but rather *who* is most important. It's not really a matter of what we should do with our time, but rather who we want to spend that time with. Who would be the audience for anything we do? For whom will our last acts be intended?

As I first began to work on this book in earnest, I happened to mention the project to the wife of one of my patients. She herself had multiple myeloma, an often-fatal form of cancer that seemed in her case to be relatively indolent. I described the premise of the book and was deflated to learn that she had just read a book exactly like mine. This wasn't a book review I wanted to hear.

After a brief exchange, though, I realized with relief that she had just read a book about "life lists," the roster of things that people have decided they want to do at some point in their lives. Not the same thing at all, I said. But she didn't agree.

"Isn't that really what your book will be about? It's about making a life list—just a very short one, right? If you have forty years left, you might have a ten-page list, but if you have a day, your list shrinks to the one item at the top."

I could see her point. So I asked her what was at the top of her life list.

She said she had always wanted to climb Mount Everest, or at least to make an attempt. She'd always wanted to do that since she visited Nepal in a year of travel after college, but family and work had intervened. If she had only a month to live, and if money and practical considerations weren't an obstacle, then yes, that's exactly what she'd want to do.

But then she became silent for a moment, staring at a point just over my left shoulder. Not meeting my gaze, exactly, though not looking away either. "But," she hesitated, "I'd want to go with my family."

She paused again, and I spent those moments of silence contemplating the vision of her entire clan being hauled up to base camp by an army of Sherpas. I assumed that she was having the same thoughts, and I expected her next sentence would be an acknowledgement that such an expedition wasn't really possible. An acknowledgement, at least, and perhaps a retraction. But her next comment surprised me.

"And especially my sister. I'd want my sister to be there." I'd recently heard about my patient's plans for the upcoming holidays, and they didn't include anyone from her sister's family. So I said I'd assumed that they weren't especially close.

They weren't close now, she said, but they had been, once. They hadn't had a falling out, exactly. But her sister wasn't as financially well off as she was, and family gatherings were awkward largely because of friction between my patient, a business owner, and her sister's husband, who had retired from a large city police force on disability and now worked part-time jobs.

We both thought about this a bit more. And she seemed to realize, I think, that if she had only a month to live, she probably wouldn't want to transport her extended family to Nepal. She didn't really want that any more than she wanted to climb Everest on her own. What she wanted, really, was to spend time with her sister.

I'd caught her, in a sense, in between two sets of goals. There were, on one hand, the wide-open "anything is possible" goals of a life list, which she hadn't yet put behind her. And on the other, the narrower goals drawn from a constrained set of possibilities—the focus of Sylvester's question to me—that she hadn't yet focused on.

Linking those two sets of goals was a question that she had answered without my asking it. What was most important to her, really, was to spend time with her sister and to bring her family back together. Strip away her dream of climbing a mountain, and family reconciliation was her implicit answer.

I'm not sure if that conversation changed the way she thought about her illness and her priorities. But it did crystallize a suspicion that I'd had about Sylvester and his question to me. He had asked me the right question, I thought, but there was another question he needed to ask first. Before he could decide how to use his time, and before anyone could help him decide how to use his time, he needed to determine who was important to him. Not what, but who.

And so that's one question that I ask my patients whenever I have a chance. Who in their lives is most important to them? Who are the people who really matter? And, thinking about my patient's wife and her sister, I also ask whether there is anyone else who is important to them. Someone who is important, or maybe even most important, who isn't part of their lives right now but who perhaps should be.

Possibility and Realism

The second question I encourage my patients to consider is what's possible. What can each of us hope to accomplish with a limited amount of time, failing health, and the demands that an illness makes on us? In other words, what could Sylvester have done with the time that he had?

Although there is, for most of us, an irreducible gap between what we'd like to accomplish and what we can accomplish, that gap need not be the evidence of failure as I originally thought it was when Sylvester posed his question. There are, in fact, two parallel questions that I've learned to ask my patients in this situation.

First, what would they like to do if they had the time, talent, and skill to do anything? That question gives me a chance to find out what drives people, what motivates them to get up every morning. It's also a chance gently to dissolve layers of protection and denial.

My patients' first responses to this question are often purposefully humble. They'd just want to spend time with their family, they say. Or they just need some time to get their affairs in order. But if I push a little, many of them, I find, catch the spirit behind the question.

What if they could do anything?

Anything?

Anything at all.

One of my patients told me that he wanted to be an astronaut. Not just an astronaut, in fact, he wanted to walk on the moon. He shrugged, smiled. But something about his smile—genuine enough, but not reflected in his eyes—warned me not to laugh.

Instead, I nodded and said I'd often wondered what it felt like to walk on the moon, and that I couldn't imagine any other experience, in our lifetime, that would have come close. I'm certain he knew this goal was a laughable one for a man in his eighties with advanced lung cancer. Nevertheless, in sharing it, he was daring me not to laugh at him. Even laughing with him would have been offensive. So I kept quiet and we both thought for a moment about what that experience must have been like.

But later, in a different conversation, we talked about what he could really do. And this is the second question I ask my patients. What do they think they can do with the time they have? What are the things they would most regret not doing?

And in a way that I can't explain but which seems true nonetheless, the first question—about what's ideal but unattainable—allows my patients to talk honestly about what is both possible and essential. It's as if that first question expands the world of what's within reach. It resets limits, making other goals seem more realistic. My patient's walk on the moon is impossible, for instance. But by comparison, a series of letters to grandchildren, or a last trip to London, or—in his case—the chance to arrange a surprise eightieth birthday party for his wife, all seem realistic.

And that, perhaps, is the secret to this pair of questions, which I've used many times since. It's a way of staking out the world of what's ideal and then rearranging the borders around what's possible. Once my patients have answered my odd question, my challenge is to help to jump from their answer—walking on the moon, learning to surf, harpooning a whale (really)—to something that they might actually achieve.

Success and Failure

As I read through these conversations and the choices that my patients make, it's difficult not to keep a running tally of what my patients accomplish. There are certainly examples that come readily to mind of those people who used the time they had left in the best possible way. The best possible way, that is, for them. These are people like Alberto or Marie or Tom, for instance, whose last acts were really pitch-perfect images of who they were and what was important to them, and how they wanted to be remembered.

And, of course, there are those like Lacy, for instance, who never really started the novel she wanted to write. And Danny should perhaps have found a better, less destructive way to recapture whatever image of himself he'd left behind him. Jose certainly didn't need to take his own life. These are tangible examples, I suppose, of last acts that could objectively be called "failures" and entered in the corresponding column of some final ledger.

But I find that these judgments of success or failure are only transient. They're washed away by a pure sense of wonder at the fragile combination of luck and timing that connects a particular set of talents and motivations with choices and opportunities. I think about all of these stories and I'm amazed, and heartened, that so many people with so little time manage to do so much.

ACKNOWLEDGMENTS

This book wouldn't have been possible without the patients I've learned from over the years, and I never would have met those patients if Janet Abrahm hadn't talked me into choosing a career in palliative care. Joan Teno and Ira Byock have been close colleagues and mentors over the years, and were liberal in the encouragement they provided in urging me to write this book. Ira deserves extra thanks for introducing me to Gail Ross and Howard Yoon, his agents and now mine. And thanks to Bob Bender, my editor at Simon & Schuster, and his assistant Johanna Li, for their restraint in dealing with the authorial equivalent of a difficult patient.

If I've learned from my patients, I've learned just as much from my friends and colleagues here at Penn, including Jason Karlawish, Jen Kapo, Joe Straton, Amy Corcoran, Lucy Pierre, Jack Coffey, and Pat Chriss. The members of my research staff have been a wonderful help, too: Kim Felsburg, Amy Pickard, Hien Lu, Dawn Smith, Fiona Paterson, Emily Trancik, Rebecca Pinnelas, Maysa De Sousa, Karen Brubaker, Megan Johnson, Leo Guercio, and Katie Wolff. I'm grateful to all of them for their comments on various drafts of the manuscript and—especially to Hien—for keeping a busy research center running on days that my mind has been elsewhere. And thanks, finally, to Sue for remembering to feed the dogs.

NOTES

Introduction: Sylvester

PAGE

17   *And nowhere is that style so vibrant:* A. Broyard, *Intoxicated by My Illness and Other Writings on Life and Death* (New York: Fawcett, 1992).

17   *"I really think you have to have":* Ibid., 63.

17   *"At the end, you're posing":* Ibid., 67.

17   *"when my doctor comes in":* Ibid., 45.

18   *"So I think we should have":* Ibid., 65.

18   *"I wanted to have":* H. Brodkey, *This Wild Darkness: The Story of My Death* (New York: Henry Holt, 1996), 84.

20   *"A hospital is full":* Broyard, *Intoxicated by My Illness,* 50.

1. Jacob: Fighting and Survival

PAGE

31   *Every year in the United States:* D. C. Angus et al., "Use of Intensive Care at the End of Life: An Epidemiologic Study," *Critical Care Medicine* 32 (2004): 638–43.

31   *Indeed, it has become masked:* M. J. Field and C. K. Cassel, eds., *Approaching Death: Improving Care at the End of Life* (Washington, D. C.: National Academy Press, 1997; D. E. Meier, R. S. Morrison, and C. K. Cassel, "Improving Palliative Care," *Annals of Internal Medicine* 127, no. 3 (1997): 225–30; *Clinical Practice Guidelines for Quality Palliative Care,* 2004, National Consensus Project for Quality Palliative Care, www.nationalconsensusproject.org.

31   *Common themes to emerge:* S. A. Payne, A. Langley-Evans, and R. Hillier, "Perceptions of a 'Good' Death: A Comparative Study of the Views of Hospice Staff and Patients," *Palliative Medicine* 10, no. 4 (1996): 307–12; P. A. Singer, D. K. Martin, and M. Kelner, "Quality End-of-Life Care: Patients' Perspectives," *Journal of the American Medical Association (JAMA)* 163, no. 8 (1999): 281; K. Steinhauser et al., "In Search of a Good Death: Observations of Patients, Families, and Providers," *Annals of Internal Medicine* 132 (2000): 825–32; K. E. Steinhauser et al., "Factors Considered Important at the End of Life by Patients, Physicians, and Other Care Providers," *JAMA* 284, no. 19 (2000): 2476–82.

32   *It has become, in my view:* S. J. Gould, "The Median Is Not the Message," *Discover* 6 (1985): 40–42.

33   *But it was then:* M. F. Greene, *Last Man Out: The Story of the Springhill Mine Disaster* (Orlando, Fla.: Harcourt, 2003).

34   *In fact, she admitted:* E. Kübler-Ross, *On Death and Dying* (New York: Macmillan, 1969), 139.

34   *Indeed, hope has become:* J. Groopman, *The Anatomy of Hope: How People Prevail in the Face of Illness* (New York: Random House, 2003).

35   *We know, for instance:* Angus et al., "Use of Intensive Care," 638–43.

35   *Patients who survive:* J. S. Turner, S. J. Briggs, and H. E. Springhorm, "Patients' Recollections of Intensive Care Unit Experiences," *Critical Care Medicine* 18 (1990): 966–68.

35   *She found that the vast majority:* T. R. Fried et al., "Understanding the Treatment Preferences of Seriously Ill Patients," *New England Journal of Medicine* 346, no. 14 (2002): 1061–66.

35   *Still, many patients do enroll:* C. Daugherty et al., "Perceptions of Cancer Patients and Their Physicians Involved in Phase I Trials," *Journal of Clinical Oncology* 13 (1995): 1062–72; K. M. Schutta and C. B. Burnett, "Factors That Influence a Patient's Decision to Participate in a Phase I Cancer Clinical Trial," *Oncology Nursing Forum* 27 (2000): 1435–38; K. Itoh et al., "Patients in Phase I Trials of Anti-Cancer Agents in Japan: Motivation, Comprehension and Expectations," *British Journal of Cancer* 76 (1997): 107–13; S. Rodenhuis et al., "Patient Motivation and Informed Consent in a Phase I Study of an Anticancer Agent," *European Journal of Cancer and Clinical Oncology* 20 (1984): 457–62.

36   *For instance, in one:* Daugherty, "Perceptions of Cancer Patients," 1062–72.

36   *Admitting defeat:* D. Casarett et al., "Improving Use of Hospice Care in the Nursing Home: A Randomized Controlled Trial," *JAMA* 294 (2005): 211–17.

37   *When the merchant brig:* D. King, *Skeletons on the Zahara* (New York: Little, Brown & Co., 2004).

37   " 'Tis enough: Ibid., 94.

38   But David Bell: D. E. Bell, "Regret in Decision Making
      Under Uncertainty," *Operations Research* 30 (1982), 961–81;
      G. Loomes and R. Sugden, "Regret Theory: An Alternative
      Theory of Rational Choice Under Uncertainty," *Economic
      Journal* 92 (1983): 805–24.

2. Danny: Parties and Celebrations

PAGE

59   *Sodom and Gomorrah:* A. Munthe, *The Story of San Michele*
      (New York: Dutton, 1930), 165.

59   *Munthe's description is a bit:* F. M. Snowden, *Naples in the
      Time of Cholera: 1884-1911* (Cambridge: Cambridge Uni-
      versity Press, 1996).

60   *That wine, shared out:* A. McKee, *Death Raft* (New York:
      Scribner, 1975).

62   *"Since I have been writing":* J. Arriens, *Welcome to Hell: Letters
      and Writings from Death Row* (Princeton: Princeton Univer-
      sity Press, 1978), 194.

65   *"You can only attend":* H. Prejean, *Dead Man Walking* (New
      York: Random House, 1993), 82.

77   *And another who wanted a winter coat:* Myra Bluebond-
      Langner, *The Private Worlds of Dying Children* (Princeton:
      Princeton University Press, 1978), 194.

3. Alberto: Reconnection and Reconcilation

PAGE

87   *In fact, in the first study:* Payne, Langley-Evans, and Hillier, "Perceptions of a 'Good' Death," 307–12.

87   *So I might tell them:* K. Lezin, *Finding Life on Death Row* (Boston: Northeastern University Press, 1999), 184.

87   *Or I might tell them about one:* J. Dwyer and K. Flynn, *102 Minutes: The Untold Story of the Fight to Survive Inside the Twin Towers* (New York: Henry Holt, 2005), 237–38.

88   *But her husband, Anthony:* S. Porter, *The Great Plague* (Phoenix Mill: Sutton Publishing Co., 1999), 40.

88   *And funerals were banned:* Ibid., 58.

89   *Perhaps the study that showed:* L. L. Carstensen and B. F. Fredrickson, "Socioemotional Selectivity in Healthy Older People and Younger People Living With the Human Immunodeficiency Virus: The Centrality of Emotion When the Future Is Constrained," *Health Psychology* 17 (1998): 1–10.

91   *We've found, for instance:* M. Collins et al., "Are Depressed Patients More Likely to Share Health Care Decisions with Others?" *Journal of Palliative Medicine,* 2004:7(4): 527–32.

91   *We've also found:* D. Casarett et al., "Making Difficult Decisions About Hospice Enrollment: What Do Patients and Families Want to Know?" *Journal of the American Geriatrics Society* 53 (2005): 249–254.

105   *That was the case:* J. Jackson, *A Furnace Afloat: The Wreck of the* Hornet *and the Harrowing 4,300 Mile Voyage of Its Survivors* (New York: Free Press, 2003).

4. Jerry: Asking Forgiveness and Making Amends

PAGE

125   *Ellen paused, Brodkey recalls:* Brodkey, *This Wild Darkness.*

136   *That information in particular:* A. Kleinman, *Patients and Healers in the Context of Culture* (Berkeley: University of California Press, 1980).

5. Marie: Revenge and Forgiveness

PAGE

151   *She agrees, but only to distract:* B. Bettelheim, *The Informed Heart* (Glencoe, Ill.: Free Press, 1960), 264–65.

152   *He salvaged from that:* J. Bardach and K. Gleeson, *Man is Wolf to Man: Surviving the Gulag* (Berkeley: University of California Press, 1998).

152   *Similar stories, incidentally:* L. Rees, *Auschwitz: A New History* (New York: Public Affairs, 2005), 116–17.

152   *Doing so, he says:* C. A. Kaplan, *Warsaw Diary of Chaim A. Kaplan* (New York: Macmillan, 1973 [orig. 1965]), 382.

152   *Indeed, an obligation to record:* P. Levi, *Survival in Auschwitz* (New York: Collier Books, 1969), 36; E. Weisel, *One Generation After* (New York: Avon, 1972), 53.

157   *He saw himself:* F. Zorn, *Mars* (New York: Knopf, 1982), 212.

158   *When plague ravaged London:* Porter, *The Great Plague.*

162   *"He wasn't willing to take part":* M. Mulvey-Roberts, ed., *Writing for Their Lives: Death Row USA* (Urbana: University of Illinois Press, 2007), 161.

6. Tom: Work and Habit

183   *Or she'd seek out:* N. D. Spingarn, *Hanging In There* (New York: Stein & Day, 1982), 151.

184   *To push those sorts:* G. Olsen, *The Deep Dark: Tragedy and Redemption in America's Richest Silver Mine* (New York: Crown, 2005), 255.

185   *But he soon found:* P. Noll, *In the Face of Death* (New York: Penguin, 1989), 57.

186   *For instance, several studies:* A. M. Arozullah et al., "The Financial Burden of Cancer: Estimates from a Study of Insured Women with Breast Cancer," *Journal of Supportive Oncology* 2, (2004): 271–78; M. Stommel, C. Given, and B. A. Given, "The Cost of Cancer Home Care to Families," *Cancer* 71 (1993): 1867–74; K. E. Covinsky et al., "Is Economic Hardship on the Families of the Seriously Ill Associated with Patient and Surrogate Care Preferences?" *Archives of Internal Medicine* 156, no. 15 (1996): 1737–41.

187   *Moreover, as a patient's family:* J. A. Hayman et al., "Estimating the Cost of Informal Caregiving for Elderly Patients with Cancer," *Journal of Clinical Oncology* 19 (2001): 3219–3225.

187   *In his memoir he concedes:* A. J. Hanlan, *An Autobiography of Dying* (Garden City, N.Y: Doubleday, 1979).

192   *Unknown to her family:* R. Powers, *Gain* (New York: Picador, 1999).

193   *He told two sociologists:* H. D. Beach and R. A. Lucas, eds., *Individual and Group Behavior in a Coal Mine Disaster* (Washington, D. C.: National Academy of Sciences, 1960), 57.

193   *In what is one:* J. Raban, *Passage to Juneau: A Sea and Its Meanings* (New York: Pantheon, 1999).

7. *Lacy: Memories and Legacies*

PAGE

210   *An article in* Time: P. Paul, "Last Wishes," *Time,* March 7, 2005.

214   *The writer Joe Fiorito:* J. Fiorito, *The Closer We Are to Dying* (New York: Picador, 2000).

214   *Jim Harrison uses:* J. Harrison, *Returning to Earth* (New York: Grove Press, 2007).

217   *Although there are several:* P. Cicchino, "Peter Cicchino's Farewell Message to Washington College of Law Students," *American University Law Review* 50 (2001): 621–26.

219   *In the Fraterville, Tennessee, mine explosion:* Coal Creek Watershed Foundation, *Coal Creek: War and Disasters,* "Fraterville Mine Disaster," www.coalcreekaml.com/Legacy4.htm.

220   *"It wasn't bad":* A. G. Breed, Associated Press wire report, January 5, 2006.

220   *"If I could impart advice":* Jackson, *A Furnace Afloat,* 138–39.

220   *But he also divulged:* Dwyer and Flynn, *102 Minutes,* 198.

223   *They understood that Julia:* Broyard, *Intoxicated by My Illness.*

224   *Peter then asked:* M. Weisman, *Intensive Care: A Family Love Story* (New York: Random House, 1982).

224   *One example that I find:* Rees, *Auschwitz.*

224   *Here Speter describes:* L. Rees, ed., Public Broadcasting Ser-

vice, "Auschwitz: Inside the Nazi State," in transcript at www.pbs.org/auschwitz/about/transcripts_5.html.

224   *The term "holophrase":* D. McNeill, *The Acquisition of Language* (New York: Harper & Row, 1970).

8. Ladislaw: Giving and Helping

PAGE

233   *Over the three years:* D. Casarett et al., "Does a Palliative-Care Clinic Have a Role in Improving End-of-Life Care?" *Journal of Palliative Medicine* 5 (2002): 387–96.

238   *"There is so much left to do":* J. Farrow, *Damien, the Leper* (New York: Sheed & Ward, 1937).

246   *Harold Brodkey's beautifully chiseled account:* Brodkey, *This Wild Darkness.*

246   *Or Anatole Broyard's lyrical account:* Broyard, *Intoxicated by My Illness.*

246   *Or Tim McLaurin's rough:* T. McLaurin, *Keeper of the Moon* (New York: Norton, 1991).

246   *There have been journalists:* Spingarn, *Hanging In There.* M. A. Lerner, *Wrestling with the Angel* (New York: Norton, 1990); S. Alsop, *Stay of Execution: A Sort of Memoir* (Philadelphia: Lippincott, 1973).

246   *And scientists like Stephen Jay Gould:* S. J. Gould, "The Median Is Not the Message," *Discover* 6 (1985): 40–42.

246   *And of course there have been teachers:* Hanlan, *An Autobiography,* 35.

246   *His goal, he chides them:* Ibid., 154.

256   *"I thought that it would":* V. Frankl, *Man's Search for Meaning* (Boston: Beacon Press, 1992 [orig. 1959]), 59–60.

9. Jose: Hopelessness and Fear

PAGE

270   *One national survey found:* D. E. Meier et al., "A National Survey of Physician-Assisted Suicide and Euthanasia in the United States," *New England Journal of Medicine* 338 (1998): 1193–201.

270   *And this figure may be:* E. J. Emanuel et al., "Attitudes and Practices of U.S. Oncologists Regarding Euthanasia and Physician-Assisted Suicide," *Annals of Internal Medicine* 133 (2000): 527–32.

271   *Anthony Black, an oncologist:* A. L. Back et al., "Physician-Assisted Suicide in Washington State: Patient Requests and Physician Responses," *JAMA* 275 (1996): 919–25.

271   *In a survey, Zeke:* E. J. Emanuel, D. L. Fairclough, and L. L. Emanuel, "Attitudes and Desires Related to Euthanasia and Physician-Assisted Suicide Among Terminally Ill Patients and Their Caregivers," *JAMA* 284 (2000): 2460–68.

271   *So the number of people:* Ibid.

272   *Diane Meier, a palliative-care physician:* D. E. Meier et al., "Characteristics of Patients Requesting and Receiving Physician-Assisted Death," *Archives of Internal Medicine* 163, no. 13 (2003): 1537–42.

273   *Bob Pearlman, a geriatrician:* R. A. Pearlman et al., "Motivations for Physician-Assisted Suicide," *Journal of General Internal Medicine* 20 (2005): 234–39.

273 *Indeed, other very carefully designed studies:* L. Ganzini et al., "Oregonians' Reasons for Requesting Physician Aid in Dying," *Archives of Internal Medicine* 169, no. 5 (2009): 489–492.

276 *On the night of August 20:* J. R. Carr, *All Brave Sailors: The Sinking of the Anglo-Saxon, August 21, 1940* (New York: Simon & Schuster, 2004).

278 *For instance, Linda Ganzini:* L. Ganzini et al., "Oregonians' Reasons."

279 *In a wonderfully elegant study:* J. R. Lunney et al., "Patterns of Functional Decline at the End of Life," *JAMA* 289, no. 18 (2003): 2387–92.

281 *He describes, for instance:* A. Donat, *The Holocaust Kingdom: A Memoir* (New York: Holt, Rinehart & Winston, 1965), 158.

282 *When Polina Melnikova hung herself:* E. Ginzburg, *Within the Whirlwind* (New York: Harvest Books, 1981), 198.

282 *Suicides of this kind:* T. Todorov, *Facing the Extreme: Moral Life in the Concentration Camps* (New York: Metropolitan Books, 1996), 63.

288 *Those who had begun:* V. Frankl, *Man's Search for Meaning.*

10. Christine: Appreciation and Wisdom

PAGE

303 *For instance, Elisabeth Kübler-Ross's stages:* Kübler-Ross, *On Death and Dying.*

304 *So over the course:* A. Heim, "Notizen über den Tod durch absturz" [Remarks on Fatal Falls], *Journal of the Swiss Alpine*

Club (1892): 327–37. Translated by Roy Kletti and reprinted in Russell Noyes and Roy Kletti, "The Experience of Dying from Falls," *Omega* 3 (1972): 45–52.

309   *Despite the fact that they:* Frankl, *Man's Search for Meaning,* 50–51.

309   *And yet these moments are:* Brodkey, *This Wild Darkness.*

316   *Someone with practical wisdom:* Aristotle, *Nicomachean Ethics,* 1141b9–14 (Englewood Cliffs, N. J.: Prentice-Hall, 1962.)

INDEX